MRCP Part 2

Best of Five Illustrated
Questions and Answers

Commissioning Editor: Ellen Green
Project Development Manager: Clive Hewat
Project Manager: Nancy Arnott/Emma Riley
Designer: Erik Bigland

MRCP Part 2

Best of Five Illustrated Questions and Answers

Huw Beynon BSc MD FRCP

Consultant Physician
Department of Rheumatology
Royal Free Hospital
London

Luke Gompels MA MRCP

Specialist Registrar Rheumatology and General Internal Medicine
Department of Rheumatology
Charing Cross Hospital
London

THIRD EDITION

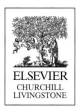

ELSEVIER
CHURCHILL
LIVINGSTONE

Edinburgh   London   New York   Oxford   Philadelphia   St Louis   Sydney   Toronto   2005

ELSEVIER
CHURCHILL
LIVINGSTONE

First edition 1991
Second edition 1998
Reprinted 2000
Reprinted 2001
Third edition 2005

ISBN 0443073317

British Library Cataloguing in Publication Data
A catalogue record for this book is available from the British Library

Library of Congress Cataloging in Publication Data
A catalog record for this book is available from the Library of Congress

Note
Knowledge and best practice in this field are constantly changing. As new research
and experience broaden our knowledge, changes in practice, treatment and drug
therapy may become necessary or appropriate. Readers are advised to check the
most current information provided (i) on procedures featured or (ii) by the
manufacturer of each product to be administered, to verify the recommended dose
or formula, the method and duration of administration, and contraindications. It is
the responsibility of the practitioner, relying on their own experience and
knowledge of the patient, to make diagnoses, to determine dosages and the best
treatment for each individual patient, and to take all appropriate safety
precautions. To the fullest extent of the law, neither the Publisher nor the Authors
assume any liability for any injury and/or damage to persons or property arising
out of or related to any use of the material contained in this book.

Printed in China

Preface

This book closely follows the new format of the MRCP examination – selecting a best answer from five. Illustrated material has been carefully chosen for two reasons: firstly to accurately reflect potential questions that may arise in the examination and secondly to optimise revision around the selected cases. For this reason answers are extended to comprehensively cover the topic area that the illustration and question stems have introduced.

Many of the cases here are based on real patient problems. It has been the experience of the authors that the knowledge and enjoyment sought from working through these cases is reflected by the sense of satisfaction achieved in improving day-to-day practice and knowhow on the wards and in the clinic – we hope that you find the same.

We gratefully acknowledge the contributions of Dr C Marguerie, Dr C Craddock, Professor van den Bogaerde and Professor Davies who were involved in previous editions of this book.

Huw Beynon
Luke Gompels

This is the magnetic resonance image of a patient who presented with confusion, ataxia and nystagmus.

a What is the diagnosis?
  1. Demyelination
  2. Thiamine deficiency
  3. CNS lymphoma
  4. Herpes simplex encephalitis
  5. Friedreich's ataxia

b What treatment would you initiate for this patient?
  1. i.v. fluconazole
  2. i.v. thiamine
  3. i.v. acyclovir
  4. i.v. methylprednisolone
  5. i.v chemotherapy

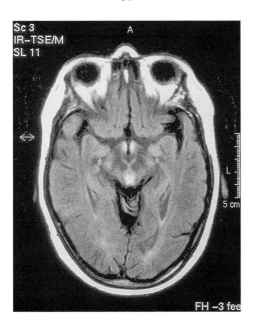

a 2. Thiamine deficiency
b 2. i.v. thiamine.

The magnetic resonance image of this patient's brain is a T1-weighted image (the CSF is dark). There are high signal areas in the periventricular areas and mamillary bodies. The clinical signs in association with these pathological changes are consistent with a diagnosis of Wernicke's encephalopathy.

Thiamine deficiency due to malnutrition, particularly in alcoholic patients, can lead to the **Wernicke–Korsakoff syndrome**. The key features of Wernicke's encephalopathy are a triad of nystagmus, ophthalmoplegia and ataxia. Other eye signs such as ptosis, abnormal pupillary reactions and altered consciousness can all be present.

A presentation with amnesia and confabulation as prominent features is termed Korsakoff's pyschosis. In these cases the clinical presentation is considered to be irreversible.

The diagnosis may be confirmed by demonstrating reduced red cell transketolase levels and raised pyruvate levels.

- Thiamine deficiency should be considered and urgently treated in alcoholic and/or malnourished patients.
- Thiamine should be given at a dose of 200–300 mg/24 h.
- Thiamine deficiency should be treated before giving intravenous glucose to prevent the risks of further depleting thiamine stores and precipitating irreversible changes.

Note:
- T1-weighted images have more contrast and fluids and CSF will appear dark, water-based tissues are mid-grey and fat-based tissues are bright. This helps most clearly to show the boundaries between tissues.
- T2-weighted images show fluid as being the brightest, with water and fat-based tissues appearing mid-grey. T2 images can be thought of as 'pathology scans': collections of abnormal fluid are brighter against the dark tissue background.

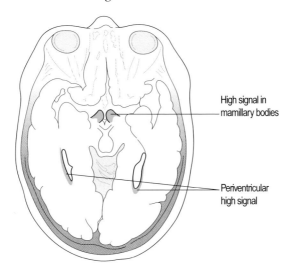

High signal in mamillary bodies

Periventricular high signal

This patient presented with a right hemiparesis. Which of the following is *not* a recognized complication of this condition?

1. Left frontal glioma
2. Left frontal cerebral abscess
3. Left middle cerebral artery embolism
4. Left frontal intracerebral bleed
5. Subarachnoid haemorrhage

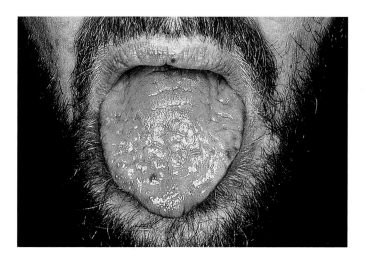

1. Left frontal glioma.

The slide shows the typical telangiectatic lesions of hereditary haemorrhagic telangiectasia (Osler–Rendu–Weber syndrome) affecting the lips and tongue.

- A telangiectasia is a cluster of dilated small blood vessels – usually capillaries and venules. It may be hereditary or acquired as in pregnancy, mitral stenosis, scleroderma and SLE.
- Small telangiectasias involve the post-capillary venules. In hereditary haemorrhagic telangiectasia, as they develop they directly involve larger venules; in the liver, lungs and brain arteriovenous malformations occur.

Hereditary haemorrhagic telangiectasia is inherited as an autosomal dominant disorder (genetic linkages established to chromosomes 9 and 12).

Clinical features include:
- Epistaxis
- Gastrointestinal haemorrhage
- Haemoptysis
- Iron deficiency anaemia
- Cerebral abscess due to pulmonary AV malformations
- Embolic stroke due to pulmonary AV malformations
- Subarachnoid haemorrhage and intracerebral bleeds
- Poor exercise tolerance due to pulmonary right-to-left shunting
- Multiple coin lesions on chest X-ray.

Anecdotally oestrogens appear to decrease the frequency of bleeds. Large pulmonary haemangiomas may be treated with embolization.

This man presented with a three-year history of tiredness and lethargy. His GP referred him to outpatients.

Which of the following can be *excluded* from the differential diagnosis?

1. Sarcoidosis
2. Sjögren's syndrome
3. Amyloidosis
4. Lymphoma
5. Mumps

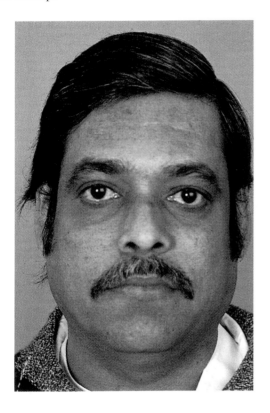

5. Mumps.

The patient has classical bilateral parotid swelling.

Mumps is a well-recognized cause of parotid swelling but can be excluded in this case on the length of the history.

The differential diagnosis of bilateral parotid swelling includes:

- Infections: mumps, bacterial parotitis
- Sarcoidosis
- Sjögren's syndrome
- AL amyloidosis
- Lymphoma
- Cirrhosis and high alcohol consumption per se
- Cystic fibrosis
- Diabetes
- Malnutrition
- Hyperlipidaemia
- Acromegaly
- Drugs, e.g. iodide, thiouracil.

Aspiration and cytological analysis of the parotids is safe in experienced hands and yielded a diagnosis of a B-cell lymphoma. The patient went on to have staging CT scans of the chest and abdomen as well as a bone marrow trephine.

Salivary gland enlargement may be accompanied by lacrimal enlargement and is a well-recognized presenting manifestation of sarcoidosis, Sjögren's syndrome and AL amyloidosis.

This young man presented with heel pain and a stiff back.
Which of the following is most likely to be positive in his case?

1. Rheumatoid factor
2. HLA B27
3. HLA DR4
4. Antinuclear antibody
5. Schirmer's test

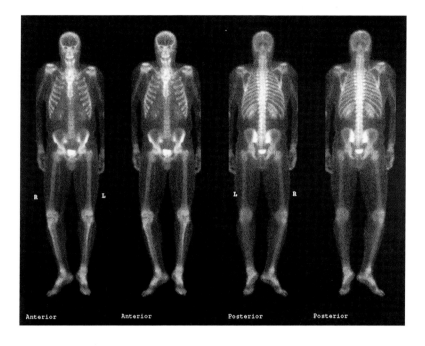

2. HLA B27.

Hot spots are visible over both sacroiliac joints and the right heel.

Ankylosing spondylitis is the most likely diagnosis in a young man with bilateral sacroiliitis and plantar fasciitis. Ankylosing spondylitis is characterized by sacroiliitis, spondylitis, inflammation of entheses and peripheral arthritis (hips, knees, shoulders and wrists). Males are affected twice as commonly as females. The MHC antigen HLA B27 is found in 96% of Caucasian cases.

Sacroiliac joints are usually the first joints affected, the patient presenting with low back pain and early morning stiffness. Radiologically sacroiliitis, which is usually symmetrical, is the hallmark of the disease. Bone scans will reveal sacroiliac inflammation before changes are visible on the plain X-ray. Involvement of the lumbar and thoracic spine follows. Erosion of the upper anterior corner of the vertebral body is the earliest radiological sign of spinal disease (the Romanus lesion); subsequent calcification causes squaring of the lumbar vertebrae. Calcification of the annulus fibrosus forms syndesmophytes, and calcification of the interspinous ligaments and longitudinal ligaments produces the typical 'bamboo spine' appearance. Restriction of chest expansion less than 2.5 cm is common in advanced cases.

Enthesitis leads to erosions and subsequent soft-tissue calcification, e.g. plantar spurs, calcification of the ischial tuberosities and the iliac crests.

Associated features of ankylosing spondylitis include:

1. Asymptomatic prostatitis (80%)
2. Anterior uveitis (25%) and conjunctivitis (20%)
3. Cardiac conduction defects, aortic incompetence
4. Pulmonary fibrosis – typically apical
5. Amyloidosis
6. Cauda equina syndrome.

Note: An enthesis is the point of insertion of a capsule, ligament or tendon into bone.

This 25-year-old female presented with a rash.
What is the most likely diagnosis?

1. Erythema marginatum
2. Secondary syphilis
3. Erythema multiforme
4. Dermatitis herpitiformis
5. Erythema nodosum

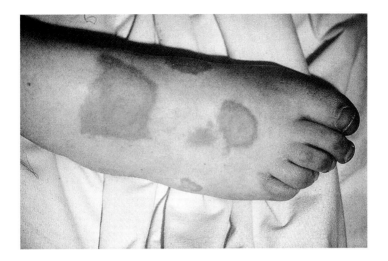

3. Erythema multiforme.

The picture shows the classical rash of **erythema multiforme**. This is an erythematous disorder characterized by annular target lesions, blistering and involvement of the mucosa can also occur. Histologically vacuolation and death of basement membrane epidermal cells is seen with vesicle formation; vasodilation and a mild lymphocytic infiltrate around superficial dermal blood vessels may also occur. This patient had a mild form of erythema multiforme, but in its most severe form, the Stevens–Johnson syndrome, a widespread vasculitis is seen. Fever, conjunctivitis, corneal scarring, epidermal necrolysis, urethritis, glomerulonephritis and pneumonitis may be seen. High-dose steroid and antibiotic therapy reduce mortality which is, however, still high.

Recognized causes of erythema multiforme include:
- Idiopathic
- Infections: herpes and mycoplasma are the most common; streptococci, typhoid, histoplasmosis, and orf are also associated
- Drugs: sulfonamides, barbiturates, sulfonylureas, salicylates and phenytoins
- Systemic diseases such as SLE and ulcerative colitis
- Carcinoma or lymphoma.

Other notes:
- Erythema marginatum is a rapidly changing figurate macular or papular erythema. It is most commonly associated with rheumatic fever. It can also be idiopathic and can occur with acute glomerulonephritis and drug reactions.
- Dermatitis herpetiformis is an intensely itchy, blistering skin condition strongly associated with a gluten-sensitive enteropathy. It can be misdiagnosed as scabies. Blisters are subepidermal. Distribution is on the extensor aspects, the scalp and scapular area. Dapsone may be used (*caution*: check that patients are not G6PD deficient, as there is a risk of provoking methaemoglobinaemia).
- Secondary syphilis may present with a papulosqamous rash which can affect the trunk, hands and feet.

Question 6

This patient has proteinuria on dipstick testing.
   What is the diagnosis?
1. Primary amyloidosis
2. Cryoglobulinaemia
3. Systemic lupus erythematosus
4. Myelofibrosis
5. Wegener's granulomatosis

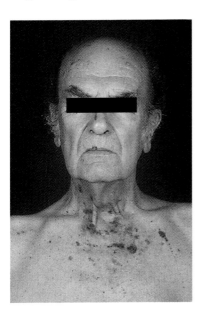

1. Primary amyloidosis.

This slide shows the typical appearance of the skin in primary amyloid (AL) with infiltration of the skin and spontaneous bruising.

Amyloid is a disorder of protein metabolism that is characterized by the extracellular deposition of abnormal protein fibrils in organs and tissues.

AL or **primary amyloidosis** is a plasma cell dyscrasia related to myeloma. Clonal plasma cells in the bone marrow produce immunoglobulins that are amyloidogenic.

AA or **secondary amyloidosis** occurs in association with:
- Chronic inflammatory disorders such as rheumatoid arthritis
- Chronic infections
- Malignancies such as Hodgkin's disease and hypernephroma.

AL amyloidosis has a wide spectrum of organ involvement. The organs most commonly involved are the kidney and the heart.
- Renal amyloidosis usually manifests as proteinuria, often resulting in the nephrotic syndrome.
- Cardiac involvement is a common presentation. A restrictive cardiomyopathy occurs in 30%.
- Autonomic and sensory neuropathies are common.
- Other features:
  — Hepatomegaly.
  — Splenomegaly is rare but functional hyposplenism is more common, occurring in 25%.
  — Vascular infiltration leads to easy bruising and the formation of ecchymoses. Spontaneous periorbital purpura can occur with sneezing.
  — Macroglossia is a classic feature.
  — Hypoadrenalism: infiltration of the adrenal glands should be investigated in the hypotensive hyponatraemic patient Both of these can occur as a result of heart failure and autonomic failure and therefore hypoadrenalism may be missed.
- A biopsy of the involved organ is usually the first diagnostic step.
- A general biopsy can be taken from the subcutaneous abdominal fat.
- Biopsies are stained with Congo red to show apple-green deposits that have positive birefringence under polarized light.
- AL is the commonest type of amyloidosis; therefore investigation should be directed towards an underlying plasma cell dyscrasia: monoclonal immunoglobulins are detected in 90% of patients with AL amyloidosis.
- If the above tests remain negative then specialized investigation for other rare mutations is required.
- Treatment is chemotherapy with autologous blood stem cell support in selected patients. This aims to achieve remission of the plasma cell dyscrasia.

AA amyloidosis presents with renal disease in most patients.
- Hepatosplenomegaly are common.
- Cardiac involvement is rare.
- Macroglossia is not a feature.

What are these findings consistent with?

1. IIIrd nerve palsy
2. IVth nerve palsy
3. VIth nerve palsy
4. Horner's syndrome
5. Wallenburg's syndrome

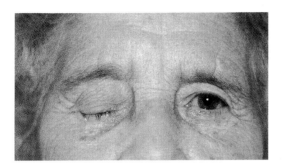

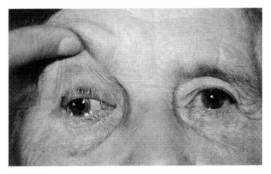

1. IIIrd nerve palsy.

The patient has a ptosis and the eye is in the 'down-and-out position'; the pupil is dilated.

- A IIIrd (oculomotor) nerve lesion causes total paralysis of the eyelid and therefore diplopia only occurs when the lid is held up. Severe diplopia occurs in all directions, except on lateral gaze to the side of the affected eye (the lateral rectus muscle supplied by the VIth nerve is intact).
- The eye is 'down' due to the depressant action of the superior oblique muscle and 'out' due to the unopposed action of the lateral rectus muscle. The pupil may be normal or dilated and fixed to light. This can help to differentiate between the various causes of a IIIrd nerve palsy. As a general rule a pupil-sparing IIIrd nerve palsy which is painless is more likely to be a 'medical' cause, diabetes being the commonest example. A painful or non-pupil-sparing palsy is more likely to have a surgical cause: aneurysms, pituitary tumours etc.

The causes of a third nerve palsy include:

1. Hypertension
2. Diabetes (typically a painless pupil-sparing IIIrd nerve palsy)
3. Multiple sclerosis
4. Aneurysm of the posterior communicating artery
5. Trauma
6. Tumours
7. Collagen disorders
8. Syphilis
9. Ophthalmoplegic migraine
10. Encephalitis
11. Parasellar neoplasms
12. Meningioma of the sphenoid wing
13. Basal meningitis
14. Carcinoma of the skull base
15. The causes of mononeuritis multiplex (this includes diabetes, malignancy, sarcoid, Churg–Strauss syndrome, rheumatoid arthritis, tuberculous leprosy, Lyme disease).

This 30-year-old female developed a rash in the second trimester of her third pregnancy.

What is the diagnosis?

1. Polymorphic eruption of pregnancy
2. Prurigo of pregnancy
3. Pemphigoid gestationis (herpes gestationis)
4. Pemphigus vulgaris
5. Herpes zoster

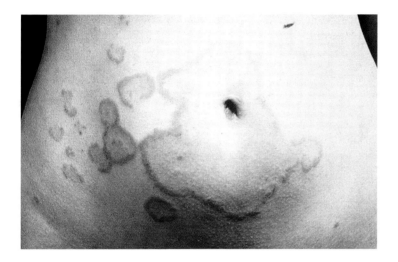

3. Pemphigoid gestationis (herpes gestationis).

The slide shows the classical periumbilical bullous lesions of pemphigoid gestationis (herpes gestationis). This is a rare, pruritic, bullous disease of pregnancy. The rash may occur during the first pregnancy but usually is seen in the second or third trimester of subsequent pregnancies. Bullous lesions develop on the hands and around the umbilicus and the mouth. Lesions usually resolve two to three weeks after delivery. The disease tends to recur with increasing severity in successive pregnancies. Exacerbations may occur premenstrually or with the oral contraceptive pill.

Treatment is with systemic corticosteroids. Histology shows that blisters form above the basement membrane; direct immunofluorescence reveals C3 and IgG deposition along the basement membrane. Placental transfer of IgG antibodies can cause a self-limiting bullous rash in the neonate.

Other notes:

- The polymorphic rash of pregnancy consists of pruritic urticated papules and plaques which are associated with severe itching. The aetiology is unknown but there is an increased incidence with progressive pregnancies.
- Prurigo of pregnancy is an eruption that occurs in the second or third trimester and consists of excoriated papules; this is also associated with intense itching.
- Pemphigus vulgaris is an intra-epidermal blistering disease that occurs predominantly in elderly patients.
- Herpes zoster is dermatomal in distribution.

This 27-year-old man presented to his GP.
What is the clinical diagnosis?

1. Acanthosis nigricans
2. Addison's disease
3. Hypothyroidism
4. Eruptive xanthomatosis
5. Tinea corporis

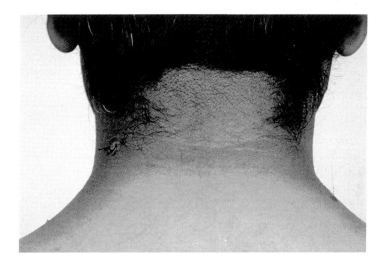

1. **Acanthosis nigricans.**

The slide demonstrates acanthosis nigricans, a velvety hyperpigmentation that most commonly appears in the flexural areas. It is most closely associated with underlying malignancy.

Recognized associations include:

1. Underlying malignancy: usually gastric adenocarcinoma, although squamous carcinoma is reported. (*Acanthosis nigricans may be seen before or after presentation with malignancy.*)
2. Obesity
3. Inherited
4. Endocrinological: diabetes mellitus, insulin resistance, lipodystrophy, Cushing's syndrome, acromegaly, polycystic ovary syndrome, hypothyroidism.

What is the most likely age range of this patient?

1. 20–30 years
2. 30–40 years
3. 40–50 years
4. 50–60 years
5. >60 years

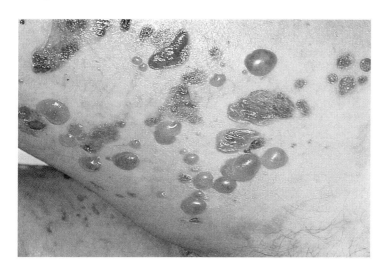

5. >60 years.

Large bullous lesions typical of the subepidermal blisters of pemphigoid are seen.

Bullous pemphigoid is the most common autoimmune blistering skin disease. It is one of the few autoimmune diseases to occur most frequently in elderly patients. 80% of patients are older than 60 years. Lesions typically consist of tense blisters occurring on either normal or erythematous skin. They are usually confined to the trunk; flexural lesions are common and oral lesions are rare. Histology demonstrates C3 and immunoglobulin deposition at the dermo-epidermal junction. Antibodies to the hemidesmosome, which are usually IgG4, are found in 70% of patients. Steroid therapy (prednisolone 0.5–1 mg/kg/day) is usually effective, and should be used for approximately six months.

Other notes:
- Benign mucosal pemphigoid (cicatrical pemphigoid) is a disorder that causes great morbidity. Subepidermal bullae occur in the mouth, conjunctiva and perianal regions. Chronic inflammation in the eye can lead to entropion and blindness.
- Pemphigus vulgaris often involves mucosa; blisters are more superficial and fragile and they occur intradermally. High-dose steroids (prednisolone 1–2 mg/kg per day) result in mortality reduction. Azathioprine or cyclophosphamide may be used in conjunction with steroids. Mortality is approximately 5%.

a What is the physical sign shown in slide A?
1. Koilonychia
2. Leukonychia
3. Beau's lines
4. Nail-fold telangiectasia
5. Paronychia

b What diagnosis encompasses signs A and B?
1. Lymphoma
2. Dercum's disease
3. Chronic iron deficiency
4. Recent chemotherapy
5. Dialysis-dependent chronic renal failure

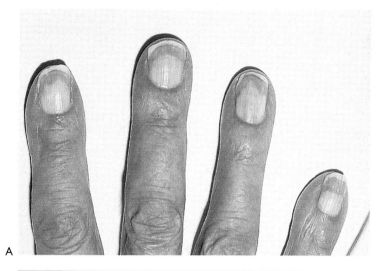

A

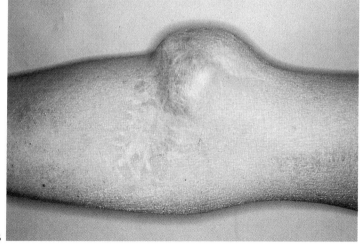

B

a 2. Leukonychia
b 5. Dialysis-dependent chronic renal failure.

Slide B shows an arteriovenous forearm fistula with local aneurysm formation.

The differential diagnosis of white nails includes:

1. Darier's disease (An autosomal dominant condition characterized by the eruption of small greasy papules, usually on the trunk, extremities and face, which coalesce to give yellow brownish sheets)
2. Renal failure
3. Hypoalbuminaemia: nephrotic syndrome; liver disease; protein-losing enteropathy
4. Arsenic/cytotoxic drugs
5. Fungal infection
6. Lymphoma
7. Malaria.

Some other conditions affecting the nail:

- Beau's lines – transverse longitudinal depressions, which occur due to severe systemic illness.
- Koilonychia – spoon-shaped nails seen in iron deficiency.
- Nail-fold telangiectasia – seen in connective tissue disorders such as scleroderma and dermatomyositis.
- Paronychia – describes inflammation and swelling around the nail-fold. This is often due to bacterial (commonly anaerobes) and fungal infections (often candida) occurring particularly in occupations where the hands get constantly wet.
- Pitting – seen in psoriasis, alopecia areata, lichen planus, eczema.

This 60-year-old Asian female has severe pain in her hip and back.
   What is the diagnosis?

1. Osteoarthritis
2. Osteomalacia
3. Osteoporosis
4. Paget's disease
5. Myeloma

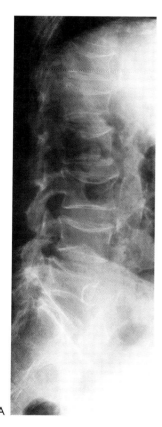

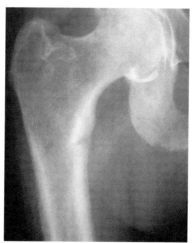

A   B

2. Osteomalacia.

The slides show the two radiological hallmarks of osteomalacia: the Looser's zone and the 'codfish spine'.

- Looser's zone refers to ribbon-like areas of defective mineralization, which may be found in almost any bone but is seen particularly in the long bones (seen here on the medial aspect of the femur), pelvis, ribs, and also around the scapulae.
- The fish spine appearance describes vertebral bodies that are often uniformly biconcave.
- In patients with osteomalacia and hypocalcaemia the radiological features of secondary hyperparathyroidism can appear with subperiosteal bone resorption, which affect the phalanges, the pubic symphysis and the outer ends of the clavicles.

Osteomalacia and rickets are characterized by defective mineralization of bone and cartilage, leading to an accumulation of unmineralized bone matrix called osteoid.

- The most common causes of osteomalacia are defects in vitamin D metabolism or, less commonly, defects in renal handling of phosphate.
- Vitamin D deficiency due to inadequate nutritional intake and reduced exposure to sunlight is more common in the immigrant Asian population.
- Characteristic symptoms are generalized bone pain and tenderness, associated with weakness of the proximal muscles. The bone pain is poorly localized and often made worse with walking.

This 45-year-old homeless man was brought into casualty drunk. What clinical diagnosis was made?

1. Thiamine deficiency
2. Septicaemia
3. Scurvy
4. Addison's disease
5. Hypothyroidism

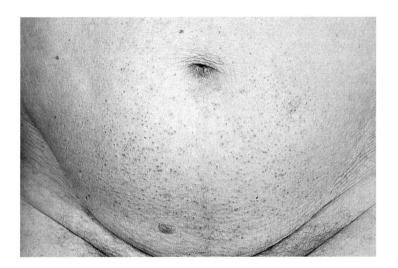

3. Scurvy.

The slide shows perifollicular haemorrhages and these are secondary to vitamin C deficiency (scurvy).

- Alcoholics are more likely to suffer from vitamin B deficiencies, but vitamin C deficiency is not uncommon in this group and is associated with a poor diet lacking in citrus fruits and green vegetables, that are the best source of vitamin C.
- Some patients with chronic diseases such as tuberculosis, smokers and users of oral contraceptives may have low vitamin C levels.
- The required daily dose of vitamin C is 60 mg, but as little as 10 mg per day is sufficient to prevent scurvy. The body stores are about 1500 mg, and increasing intake dramatically does not substantially increase serum levels or stores.
- Vitamin C is an antioxidant, enhances iron absorption, and is important in collagen hydroxylation.

Typical clinical features of ascorbic acid deficiency include:
- Lassitude, irritability and cognitive impairment
- Perifollicular skin haemorrhage and hyperkeratosis
- Alopecia, coiled fractured corkscrew hair
- Swollen haemorrhagic gums
- Haemorrhage into bone, giving a periosteal reaction
- Subconjunctival haemorrhage
- Intracerebral haemorrhage.

Which of the following is this condition *not* associated with?

1. Down's syndrome
2. Hashimoto's thyroiditis
3. Vitiligo
4. Tinea capitis
5. Spontaneous recovery

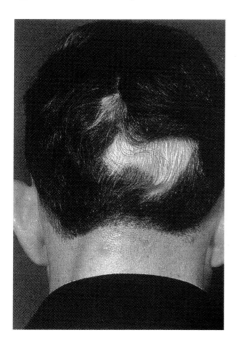

4. Tinea capitis.

The slide shows the typical appearance of alopecia areata. The hair loss is not associated with any appreciable abnormality in the underlying skin.

- Spontaneous recovery can occur in uncomplicated cases.
- A family history of other autoimmune disorders such as Hashimoto's thyroiditis and diabetes mellitus is common.
- Vitiligo is associated in 4% of cases (and there is a positive family history of alopecia in 10% of cases presenting with vitiligo).
- Histologically there is a T-helper cell lymphocytic infiltrate around the hair follicles. Unlike other autoimmune disorders, there is no permanent destruction of the target organ and the hair may regrow.
- The condition is commoner in Down's syndrome, occurring in 6% (and subjects often have alopecia universalis).
- 'Explanation mark' hairs may be present (these are short stumps of hair where the proximal portion nearest the scalp is thin and depigmented).

Note:
- *Alopecia areata* refers to one or many bald spots.
- If it affects the entire scalp then it is called *alopecia totalis*.
- If the entire body is affected then it is referred to as *alopecia universalis*.

Tinea capitis is a superficial fungal infection that leads to alopecia, leaving the surface of the skin scaly and sometimes inflamed. Small stubs of hair – 'black dots' – may be scattered in the area. Systemic antifungals are required to treat this and griseofulvin is the treatment of choice.

Scarring alopecia occurs in any disorder where there is severe inflammation of the dermis and subsequent scar tissue formation leading to permanent loss of the hair follicles.

Skin conditions that can cause scarring alopecia include:
- Lichen planus
- Scleroderma
- Discoid lupus erythematosus.

Organ-specific autoimmune disorders include (from the head down):
- Myxoedema
- Hashimoto's thyroiditis
- Graves' disease
- Idiopathic hypoparathyroidism
- Fibrosing alveolitis
- Pernicious anaemia
- Atrophic gastritis
- Diabetes mellitus
- Chronic active hepatitis
- Primary biliary cirrhosis
- Renal tubular acidosis
- Addison's disease
- Premature ovarian failure.

This man complains of low back pain and his GP has documented glycosuria in the presence of a normal blood glucose level.
What is the diagnosis?

1. Cystinosis
2. Haemochromatosis
3. Wilson's disease
4. Alkaptonuria
5. Galactosaemia

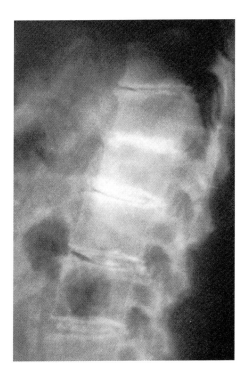

4. Alkaptonuria.

The slide shows narrowed, calcified intervertebral discs with minimal osteophyte formation.

Alkaptonuria (ochronosis) is an autosomal recessive deficiency of the enzyme homogentisic acid oxidase, which results in excess homogentisic acid accumulating in the blood, tissues and urine. Oxidation and polymerization of homogentisic acid leads to the deposition of a black pigment called alkapton in the connective tissue of the joints, intervertebral discs, sclerae, ears, nose, trachea and large vessels. The majority of patients present in middle age with back pain and stiffness. Degenerative arthritis of the knees, hips and shoulders is also common. The condition is compatible with a normal life-span and treatment is aimed at relieving symptoms.

Alkapton deposition in the ears and eyes aids the diagnosis. The urine will turn dark on standing; however, the change is often protracted unless the process is speeded up by alkalinization of the urine. Urine chromatography confirms the diagnosis. X-ray changes typically show narrowed, calcified intervertebral discs with minimal osteophyte formation. The interspinous ligament does not calcify and the sacroiliac joints are unaffected.

The reported glycosuria is a false positive Clinitest result. Homogentisic acid is a reducing substance and, as such, like all reducing substances, will give a positive result with Clinitest tablets; it will not, however, give a positive reaction with Clinistix that contains the enzyme glucose oxidase and is therefore specific for glucose.

Other notes:
- Patients with haemochromatosis develop chondrocalcinosis (calcification of the cartilage). The affected joints also show loss of joint space and subchondral cysts. The most commonly affected joints are the wrists, metacarpophalangeal joints, elbows, shoulders and knees.

This patient presented with polyuria and abdominal pain.
What is the diagnosis?

1. Multiple myeloma
2. Hypothyroidism
3. Hyperparathyroidism
4. Acute intermittent porphyria
5. Vitamin B_{12} deficiency

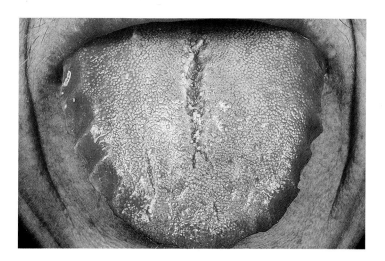

1. Multiple myeloma.

Multiple myeloma has been complicated by primary AL amyloid and macroglossia. The polyuria and abdominal pain are due to myeloma-induced hypercalcaemia.

Macroglossia is a resting tongue that protrudes beyong the teeth. It is a frequent finding in patients with primary (AL) amyloidosis. Imprints of the patient's teeth can be seen around the tongue edges.

Other conditions associated with macroglossia include:

- Amyloidosis
- Acromegaly
- Hypothyroidism (in children)
- Lymphoma
- Chronic infections: TB, syphilis.

Other notes:

- Vitamin B_{12}/folate deficiency leads to glossitis: a beefy red tongue
- In patients with Down's Syndrome relative enlargement of the tongue secondary to a small mandible is common.

This patient presented with bilateral wrist pain.

Which of the following tests would be most useful in achieving a diagnosis?

1. Nerve conduction studies
2. Muscle biopsy
3. Chest X-ray
4. Pulmonary function tests
5. β-hCG

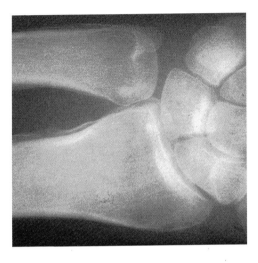

3. Chest X-ray.

This is the typical appearance of **hypertrophic pulmonary osteoarthropathy (HPOA)**. There is subperiosteal new bone formation along the diaphyses of the radius and ulna and similar changes would be expected in the tibia and fibula. HPOA is often accompanied by clubbing and an arthritis affecting the wrists and ankles.

It is most commonly associated with:
- Squamous carcinoma of the lung
- Pleural mesothelioma
- Rarely: pleural fibromas, intrapulmonary sepsis, cyanotic congenital heart disease and β-hCG-secreting tumours such as teratomas or trophoblastic tumours. (It may then also be associated with gynaecomastia.)

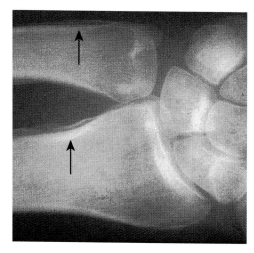

This female was investigated for persistent proteinuria and mild hypertension. A renal biopsy was performed.

Which of the following would you expect the histology to show?

1. Minimal-change glomerulonephritis
2. Membranous glomerulonephritis
3. Focal glomerulosclerosis
4. Mesangiocapillary glomerulonephritis type I
5. Mesangiocapillary glomerulonephritis type II

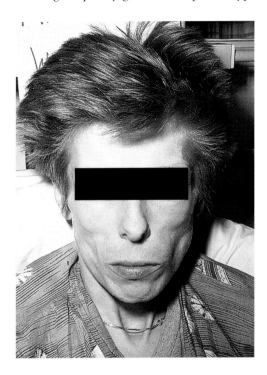

5. Mesangiocapillary glomerulonephritis type II.

This slide shows the classical appearance of facial lipodystrophy and there is a well-recognized association with mesangiocapillary glomerulonephritis type II.

Two main types of mesangiocapillary (membranoproliferative) glomerulonephritis are recognized: both have mesangial cell proliferation, diffuse thickening of the glomerular capillary walls and on electron microscopy electron dense deposits in the capillary basement membrane.

- Type I has subendothelial deposits of complement and immunoglobulin. Both C3 and C4 levels are reduced. When occurring secondary to cryoglobulinaemia it is strongly associated with hepatitis C infection.
- Type II is characterized by intramembranous deposits of electron-dense material (dense membrane deposit disease). C3 is found along the capillary loops but unlike type I no immunoglobulins are found. An autoantibody – the C3 nephritic factor – is found in 70%. This stabilizes C3bBb (the alternative complement pathway convertase enzyme), allowing uncontrolled activation of the alternative pathway, leading to low levels of C3, factor B and properdin but normal C4. It usually presents with an acute nephritis or with recurrent macroscopic haematuria.

Mesangiocapillary glomerulonephritis usually presents as a nephritic or nephrotic illness. The natural history is one of gradual deterioration to end-stage renal failure over a 10-year period.

Other causes of partial lipodystrophy:
- HIV (both directly and as a consequence of therapy)
- Localized scleroderma
- Chronic relapsing panniculitis
- Subcutaneous insulin injections.

This 30-year-old man presented with a swollen leg.
   What is the diagnosis?

1. Systemic lupus erythematosus
2. Reiter's syndrome
3. Lymphogranuloma venereum
4. Crohn's disease
5. Behçet's syndrome

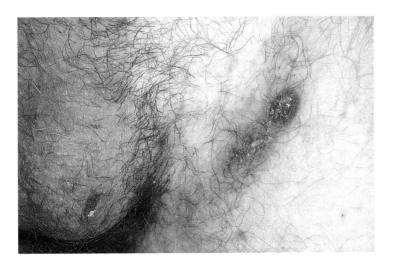

5. Behçet's syndrome.

Behçet's syndrome is a rare multisystem vasculitic disorder that affects males more commonly than females.

- The syndrome is more common in patients from Turkey, Japan, Greece and the Middle East.
- Behçet originally described a triad of recurrent oral ulceration, genital ulcers and iritis. A number of other clinical features have now been added.
- Diagnosis requires the presence of recurrent oral ulcers (minor aphthous/major aphthous or herpetiform ulcers that have recurred at least three times in a one-year period) plus any two of the following four:
  i)   Genital ulceration: ulcers or scarring
  ii)   Eye lesions: anterior or posterior uveitis; retinal vasculitis
  iii) Skin lesions: erythema nodosum; pseudofolliculitis; papulopustular lesions; or acneiform nodules
  iv)   Positive pathergy (the development of skin pustules at venepuncture points).

Other clinical features include: fever and malaise; episcleritis; papilloedema; optic atrophy; polyarthritis; arterial and venous thrombosis and localized aneurysms; diarrhoea, abdominal pain and colonic ulcers; brain stem syndromes, organic confusional states, meningitis and myelitis; pericarditis.

- Biopsies show a non-specific necrotizing small-vessel vasculitis.
- The ESR is raised; a mild anaemia is common and circulating immune complexes may be detected.
- In patients with Behçet's syndrome HLA B12 has been linked to recurrent oral ulcers and HLA B51 with ocular disease.
- Treatment is unsatisfactory, but corticosteroids and colchicine have been used with varying degrees of success.

The differential diagnosis of oral and genital ulcers is:

1. Behçet's syndrome
2. Reiter's syndrome
3. Crohn's disease
4. Pemphigus vulgaris
5. Syphilis
6. Herpes infections and HIV
7. Erythema multiforme
8. Strachan's syndrome (orogenital ulcers/sensory neuropathy/amblyopia – aetiology unknown).

What is the diagnosis?

1. Basal cell carcinoma
2. Keratocanthoma
3. Squamous cell carcinoma
4. Seborrhoeic keratosis
5. Fibrous papule

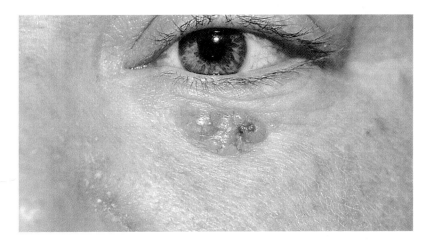

1. Basal cell carcinoma.

This shows the typical appearances of a basal cell carcinoma:

- It has a pearly translucent appearance and a central depressed area with a small amount of ulceration and a raised rolled border.
- There are telangectasia in the lesion.
- They occur more frequently on sun-exposed skin.
- It is the most common cutaneous malignancy and almost never metastasizes but invades locally.
- The major types of basal cell carcinoma are nodular and superficial spreading. The differential diagnosis depends on the type:

	Typical appearance	Differential
Nodular (the most common)	Typically slow-growing lesions. Appear translucent or pearly and demonstrate telangiectasia. Can break down into a nodulo-ulcerative pattern.	Squamous cell carcinoma, sebaceous hyperplasia, fibrous papule of the nose, non-pigmented naevus.
Superficial spreading	Thin lesions, erythematous, slow-growing plaques.	Dermatitis, psoriasis and Bowen's disease (squamous carcinoma in situ).

- Other forms include a morpheaform or sclerosing type of infiltrative lesion and rarely they can be a pigmented variation.

Other disorders:

- Fibrous papule: this is an idiopathic flesh-coloured papule that occurs on the nose in older individuals and is usually asymptomatic, but can cause concern that it may represent a basal cell carcinoma. No treatment is needed aside for cosmetic reasons.
- Squamous carcinoma: this is a malignant neoplasm of keratinocytes that is locally invasive and has the potential to metastasize. The typical appearance is of a hard papule or nodule that is erythematous or flesh coloured, smooth, scaling or crusted. The differential diagnosis includes keratoacanthoma, actinic keratosis, wart, basal cell carcinoma and seborrheic keratosis. Local excision is required, with larger lesions requiring possible block dissection and radiotherapy.
- Keratoacanthoma: this is a rapidly growing epidermal neoplasm. It is a dome-shaped, flesh-coloured nodule that has rolled borders and a central keratin plug. Lesions often disappear over a 6- to 12-month period.
- Seborrhoeic keratosis: this is a benign lesion of the epidermis, usually appearing during middle age. Unless irritated they are usually asymptomatic. They are typically well demarcated, slightly scaling, greasy appearing, tan to dark brown, pasted on papules and plaques.

What is the clinical diagnosis?

1. Pretibial myxoedema
2. Ichthyosis
3. Tylosis
4. Deliberate self-harm
5. Eczema

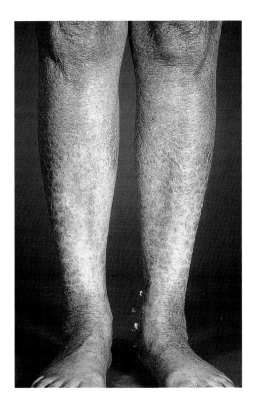

2. Ichthyosis.

The skin is rough, dry and hyperkeratotic and has the appearance of fish-like scales.

The condition may be inherited (accounting for most cases) or associated with either metabolic abnormalities or malignancy.

Inherited types include:

- Ichthyosis vulgaris
  — (autosomal dominant inheritance) Spares flexural aspects, present from childhood.
- X-linked ichthyosis
  — present from birth over trunk.
- Lamellar ichthyosis
  — (autosomal recessive inheritance) Affects whole body. Present from birth and is associated with ectropion.

Secondary causes of ichthyosis include:

- Metabolic:
  — Refsum's disease: a disorder of lipid metabolism, autosomal recessive inheritance resulting in the accumulation of phytanic acid, leading to a mixed motor and sensory polyneuropathy, cerebellar ataxia, pigmentary degeneration of the retina (retinitis pigmentosa), sensorineural deafness and cerebellar ataxia.
- Malignancy:
  — Hodgkin's disease
  — Multiple myeloma
  — Breast cancer.

Which form of hyperlipidaemia is this abnormality most commonly associated with?

1. Type IIa
2. Type III
3. Type IIb
4. Type I
5. Type IV

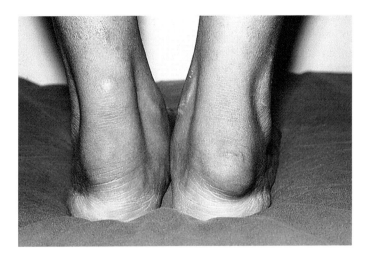

1. Type IIa hypercholesterolaemia.

The slide shows tendon xanthomas over the Achilles tendon.

This is the clinical hallmark of familial hypercholesterolaemia (WHO type IIa).

- The most common sites to find xanthomata are in the tendons overlying the knuckles and as seen here in the Achilles tendons. They can also be seen in other extensor tendons. Subperiosteal xanthomata are also commonly present on the upper tibia and the patellar tendon inserts. Patients frequently also present with corneal arcus.
- Type IIa hypercholesterolaemia is characterized by raised low-density lipoprotein levels (LDL), caused by a deficiency of LDL receptors on cell surfaces.
- Familial hypercholesterolaemia is inherited in an autosomal dominant fashion.
- Early-onset ischaemic heart disease is the commonest mode of presentation and 50% of untreated heterozygous males will have ischaemic heart disease by the age of 50 (age 60 in females). The average life-span for untreated homozygotes is 20 years.

Type	Lipoprotein increased	Lipids increased	Clinical features	Comments
I	Chylomicrons	Triglycerides	Eruptive xanthomata Abdominal pain Pancreatitis Lipaemia retinalis	Very rare
IIa	LDL	Cholesterol	Tendon xanthomata in familial form Also corneal arcus and polyarthritis	Common IHD in 50% of males by 50*
IIb	LDL and VLDL	Cholesterol and triglycerides	Increased incidence of IHD for any given level of cholesterol	Common
III	Beta-VLDL (=IDL and chylomicron elements)	Cholesterol and triglycerides	Palmar xanthomata IHD and peripheral vascular disease	Uncommon Often associated with obesity, diabetes and high alcohol intake
IV	VLDL	Triglycerides	IHD and peripheral vascular disease Eruptive xanthomatosis Lipaemia retinalis	Common Often associated with obesity, diabetes and high alcohol intake
V	Chylomicrons and VLDL	Cholesterol and triglycerides	Liable to develop pancreatitis	Uncommon Can be associated with excessive alcohol intake and diabetes

*A proportion of type IIa patients have heterozygous monogenic familial hypercholesterolaemia, as in this case.

This 35-year-old lady presented with sore and weeping arm-pits. There was no significant past medical history and she was systemically well.
What is the likely diagnosis?

1. Tuberculous lymphadenitis
2. Cat-scratch fever
3. Hidradenitis suppurativa
4. Acne rosacea
5. Miliaria

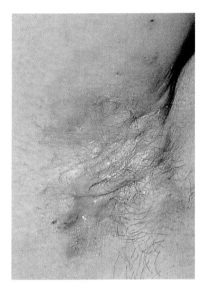

3. Hidradenitis suppurativa.

The slide shows the classical appearance of hidradenitis suppurativa. This is a chronic suppurative infection of the apocrine glands which causes multiple tender papules and pustules, leading to persistent sinus formation. Antistaphylococcal antibiotics are often effective but may need to be taken on a long-term basis. The disease is often persistent and sometimes recourse to surgery is necessary.

Other notes:

- Miliaria is a result of sweat duct blockage due to overhydrated keratin. The clinical features are itching, small vesicles, redness and papules. It is seen in hot and humid climates and resolves on returning to cooler regions.
- Acne rosacea is characterized by diffuse facial erythema, papules and pustules. The skin looks tense and shiny and telangiectasia are often present. There are no comedones or scars, which distinguishes it from acne vulgaris.
- Cat-scratch disease is characterized by regional lymphadenopathy after a cat scratch. Affected nodes are often tender and occasionally ulcerate. The underlying organism is *Bartonella henselae.*

How is this patient likely to have presented?

1. Collapse
2. Acute severe chest pain radiating to the back
3. With erythema nodosum and iritis
4. Fever, shortness of breath and purulent sputum
5. Weight loss and haemoptysis

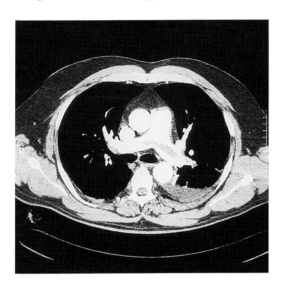

1. Collapse.

This contrast CT image shows a saddle pulmonary embolus. There is a large filling defect in the contrast-filled pulmonary artery. With such massive blockage of the pulmonary circulation this patient is likely to have presented with collapse associated with an acute onset of breathlessness.

Patients who have had a massive pulmonary embolism are equally breathless sitting upright or lying flat (contrasting with patients presenting with left ventricular failure).

Auscultation may be normal. Hypotension may be marked and pulsus paradoxus may be present. Later the embolus may disintegrate, resulting in pleuritic chest pain, a pleural rub and a blood-stained pleural effusion.

An acute major pulmonary embolus is an indication for thrombolytic therapy and in some cases a pulmonary embolectomy may be attempted.

How may this patient have presented?

1. Weight loss and change of bowel habit
2. With obstructive jaundice
3. Severe chest and abdominal pain and renal failure
4. Fever and renal angle tenderness
5. Pain on straightening the leg

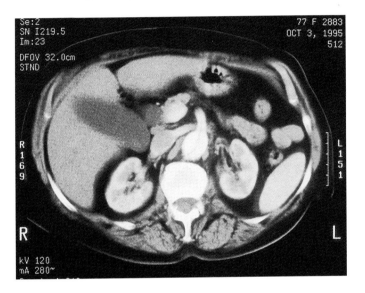

3. Severe chest and abdominal pain and renal failure.

This slide shows dissection of the aorta and the 'tennis ball' sign.

A dissection of the descending thoracic aorta may extend into the abdominal area and involve all of its major branches, thus being associated with the classical history of severe interscapular pain and acute renal failure, mesenteric ischaemia or ischaemia of the lower limbs.

Other presentations and their associated possible radiological diagnoses:

Weight loss and change of bowel habit	Suggests a large bowel tumour may be present. There is no evidence of contrast in the bowel in this study.
With obstructive jaundice	Think of hepatic metastases or a head of pancreas lesion.
Fever and renal angle tenderness	Suggests pyelonephritis, consider a renal collection.
Pain on straightening the leg	A psoas abscess may be present.

This 45-year-old Caucasian woman was found to have mild derangement of liver function on routine biochemistry. She had presented to her GP with lethargy. She gives a long history of photosensitivity and blistering over the preceding 10 years.

Which of the following drugs may improve her photosensitivity?

1. Chlorpromazine
2. Nicotinamide
3. Chloroquine
4. Pyridoxine
5. Chlorpropamide

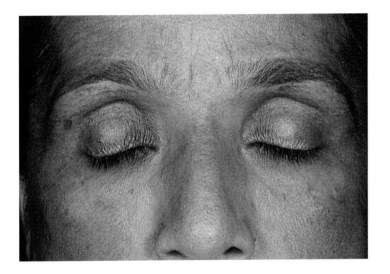

3. Chloroquine.

The patient has hyperpigmentation of her eyelids and forehead with some scarring of her skin. The rash is typically found on sun-exposed areas.
The diagnosis is **porphyria cutanea tarda (PCT)**:

- It may be familial, sporadic or associated with toxins such as hexachlorobenzene.
- The enzyme defect is uroporphyrinogen decarboxylase, which is diagnosed in the familial form by testing the enzyme in red blood cells. The sporadic and toxic forms only show the enzyme defect in the liver.
- Alcohol ingestion, intake of iron or oestrogen exposure may precipitate this disease. Uroporphyrins and coproporphyrins are found in the urine, but uroporphyrin to coproporphyrin ratio is high in PCT.
- PCT is the commonest form of porphyria in the UK. It is more common in men and patients usually present in their thirties.
- Fatty liver and mildly deranged liver function tests are common but cirrhosis is only found in 10% of patients.
- Neurological signs are not found and cutaneous features include photosensitivity, blistering, pigmentation, and depigmentation, hirsuitism, scarring, thickening and milia.
- Management includes avoidance of alcohol, oestrogen-containing compounds and direct sunlight.
- Phlebotomy can improve the condition and chloroquine 250 mg three times a week may help.

This 50-year-old man complains of marked pruritus.
What is the diagnosis?

1. Chronic urticaria
2. Carcinoid syndrome
3. Mycosis fungoides
4. Erythema ab igne
5. Acanthosis nigrans

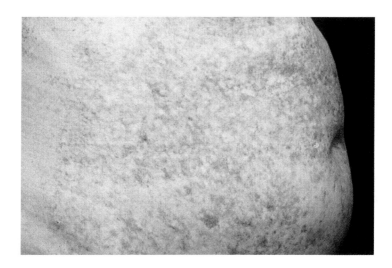

3. Mycosis fungoides.

The slide shows the appearance of poikiloderma atrophicans vasculare.

Mycosis fungoides is a cutaneous T-cell lymphoma, which typically presents in the fourth or fifth decade.

- Mycosis fungoides may be classified by stage. Poikiloderma atrophicans vasculare is the early pre-malignant stage characterized by erythema, reticulate pigmentation, telangiectasia and atrophy. Some early lesions resemble a non-specific eczematous rash. The disease may progress slowly, over 10–20 years, to an infiltrative malignant stage with multiple indurated plaques. Eventually large bluish nodules develop, which may ulcerate and discharge. Finally dissemination occurs; large numbers of mycosis fungoides cells appear in the blood and there may be lymphadenopathy and hepatosplenomegaly.
- Skin biopsies reveal mycosis fungoides cells (Sézary cells), T-lymphocytes and other inflammatory cells in the dermis. As the disease advances these cells are also seen in the epidermis, where they constitute the microabscesses of Pautrier.
- Topical steroids, topical nitrogen mustard and PUVA have been used to treat early pre-infiltrative stages; superficial X-ray therapy and chemotherapeutic agents such as methotrexate or cyclophosphamide have been used for later stages of the disease.

Sézary syndrome is a form of cutaneous T-cell lymphoma characterized by the triad of erythroderma, lymphadenopathy and atypical circulating mononuclear cells (Sézary cells).

This bone marrow transplant recipient has presented with the complication shown below.

What is the diagnosis?

1. Molloscum contagiosum
2. Psoriasis
3. Viral warts
4. Lichen planus
5. Sarcoidosis

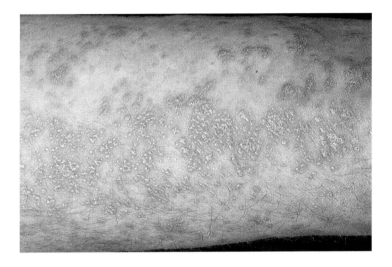

4. Lichen planus.

- The patient has developed **lichen planus** and the slide shows typical flat-topped purple polygonal papules. Lichen planus usually starts on the flexor aspect of the wrist; lesions on the shins may coalesce, forming hypertrophic plaques. The fine, white, lace-like lesions visible on the surface of some papules are called Wickham's striae. Mucosal lesions occur in up to 70% of cases; they are usually visible opposite the premolar teeth; in severe cases ulceration can occur.
- Lichen planus, along with psoriasis and viral warts, exhibits the Koebner phenomenon (further lesions develop at sites of trauma).

The lesions of lichen planus are said to be: **p**lentiful, **p**ruritic, **p**olygonal, **p**olished, **p**urple, **p**lanar **p**apules.

- Histology of lichen planus lesions shows a heavy lymphocytic infiltrate adjacent to the lower surface of the epidermis, liquefactive degeneration of the epidermal basement membrane and saw-toothing of the rete ridges. Other features include hyperkeratosis and an increase in the epidermal granular layer. Pathogenesis is poorly understood, although an immunological mechanism seems likely.
- Recognized causes of lichen planus include:
  — Graft versus host disease following bone marrow transplant
  — Drugs, e.g. gold, penicillamine, antimalarials, sulfonylureas, beta-blockers, thiazides, methyldopa
  — Chemicals (e.g. colour developers).
- Topical steroids, often in combination with polythene occlusion, are the treatment of choice for mild cases; oral steroids are used in severe cases. Metronidazole is effective for ulcerative oral lichen planus.

This 17-year-old boy has presented with a painful lump on the head. He was systemically well. (Clinical examination showed a firm lump.)

Routine chest X-ray was normal. His full blood count, liver function tests, serum calcium and urea and electrolytes were all normal. His skull X-ray is shown.

The most likely diagnosis is:

1. Multiple myeloma
2. Hyperparathyroidism
3. Osteomyelitis
4. Langerhans cell histiocytosis
5. Osteomalacia

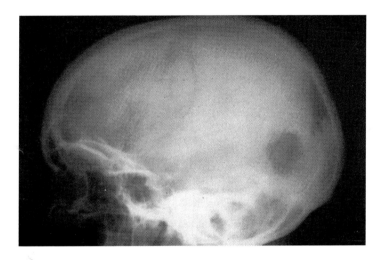

4. Langerhans cell histiocytosis.

The differential diagnosis of discrete translucencies on a skull X-ray include:

- Multiple myeloma
- Hyperparathyroidism
- Metastatic deposits
- Langerhans cell histiocytosis
- Sarcoidosis
- Leukaemia
- Sickle cell disease
- Congenital cranial lacunae.

Langerhans cell histiocytosis most commonly presents with painful bone swelling. Virtually any bone can be affected – the skull is one of the commonest. Adjacent soft tissues can be involved and there may be ulceration of the overlying skin. X-rays show the classical well-defined osteolytic lesion as seen here. A sclerotic margin is evidence of healing but raises the differential diagnosis of malignancy or osteomyelitis.

- This is a disorder characterized by the proliferation of epidermal Langerhans cells. These cells migrate from the epidermis to the dermis and other organs, where they proliferate, secrete cytokines and cause end-organ damage. It appears to be a clonal disorder but whether it represents a form of cancer is open to dispute.
- It has a peak age of onset of 1–2 years, with a range from birth to old age.
- Males are affected twice as commonly as females.
- The clinical spectrum is wide and the prognosis depends on the extent and distribution of the disease.
- Multisystem involvement with bone marrow and liver involvement may be associated with significant mortality.
- Single organ involvement is often accompanied by spontaneous resolution, although lung fibrosis may occur.
- Single organ disease occurs in the following decreasing order of frequency:
    1. Bone as above
    2. Skin resembles seborrhoeic eczema
    3. Reticuloendothelial: lymphadenopathy, splenomegaly
    4. Ears: otitis externa, aural polyps
    5. Peripheral blood: anaemia, pancytopenia
    6. Liver: hepatomegaly/low albumin, elevated PT
    7. Lungs: fibrosis with honeycombing/ pneumothoraces (localized lung disease occurs predominantly in smokers)
    8. CNS: cranial diabetes insipidus.
- The diagnosis is confirmed by biopsy.
- Single osteolytic lesions will often undergo spontaneous resolution.
- Occasionally radiotherapy is required for expanding bone lesions.
- For symptomatic systemic disease corticosteroids and cytotoxics may be necessary.

Question 30

What is the diagnosis?

1. Peutz–Jeghers syndrome
2. Addison's disease
3. Hereditary haemorrhagic telangectasia
4. Familial adenomatous polyposis
5. Gardner's syndrome

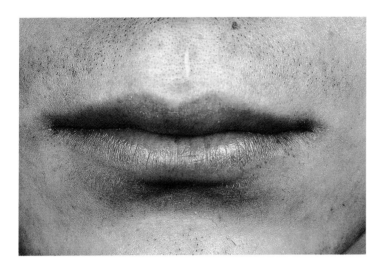

1. **Peutz–Jeghers syndrome.**

The slide shows typical small perioral pigmented macules extending beyond the margins of the lips, consistent with a diagnosis of Peutz–Jeghers syndrome.

- This is an autosomal dominant condition.
- Multiple polyps (hamartomas) occur throughout the small intestine.
- Complications include intussusception, anaemia and, less commonly, malignant transformation.
- Pigmentation can also occur on the buccal mucosa but never on the tongue.

Other notes:

- Addison's disease can also be associated with buccal pigmentation in addition to the general pigmentation found, which is more marked in skin creases, around the nipples and at pressure points.
- Familial adenomatous polyposis (FAP) is mainly an autosomal dominant condition, with the defect localized to the APC gene on chromosome 5q21 (10% of individuals have new mutations). The condition leads to the formation of multiple polyps in the colon. These appear between the age of 10 and 35 years. Patients are screened annually and require a prophylactic colectomy, otherwise the development of carcinoma is almost inevitable.
- Gardner's syndrome is a variant of FAP in which affected members develop extraintestinal soft-tissue tumours (osteomas, lipomas and dermoid tumours) associated with abnormal pigmentation of the fundi.

This patient has a long history of painless diarrhoea. He complains of bulky stools that are difficult to flush. His GP has diagnosed type II diabetes and commenced him on metformin.

What is the diagnosis?

1. Coeliac disease
2. Giardiasis
3. Short gut syndrome
4. Chronic pancreatitis
5. Metformin intolerance

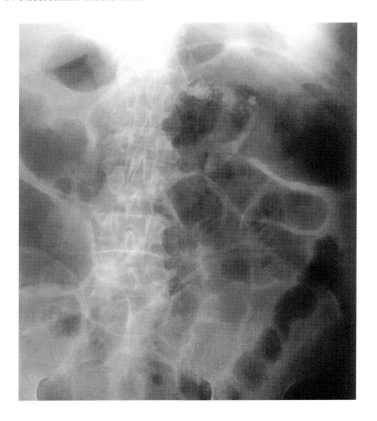

4. Chronic pancreatitis.

This plain abdominal X-ray shows calcification in the pancreas. This has occurred as a result of chronic pancreatitis.

This can present insidiously with abdominal pain, diarrhoea, steatorrhoea and consequent weight loss. Patients often develop secondary diabetes.

Chronic alcoholism is the commonest cause in adults (cystic fibrosis being the commonest in children).

The most sensitive test to make the diagnosis is the hormone stimulation test. This, however, requires intestinal intubation.

Ultrasonography and CT allow early detection of calcification and can detect duct dilatation, the presence of obstructing masses and pseudocysts.

The most important management steps are to provide pancreatic enzyme replacements. Abstinence from alcohol and a low-fat diet are also recommended.

Other causes of pancreatic calcification include:
- Idiopathic pancreatitis
- Trauma
- Islet cell tumours
- Hypercalcaemia
- Familial pancreatitis
- Malnutrition.

Note: Metformin can be associated with diarrhoea on initiation of treatment. It is therefore recommended that the dose is incrementally increased.

What is the unifying diagnosis?

1. Carcinoma of head of pancreas
2. Crohn's disease
3. Ulcerative colitis
4. Chronic active hepatitis
5. Secondary syphilis

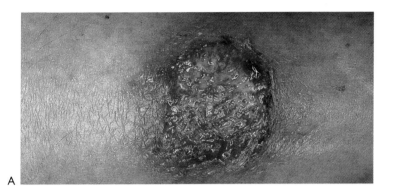

A

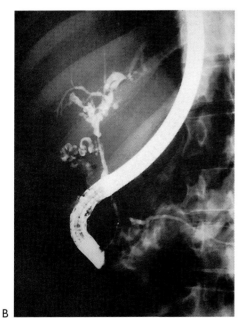

B

3. Ulcerative colitis.

- Slide A shows pyoderma gangrenosum; there is a large ulcer with a necrotic base and overhanging purple edge.
- Slide B is of an ERCP (endoscopic retrograde cholangiopancreatograph). This shows the classical appearance of sclerosing cholangitis with narrowing and bead-like dilations of the biliary tree.

Ulcerative colitis is a chronic inflammatory condition affecting the mucosa of the colon and rectum. Active disease is associated with fever, bloody diarrhoea, weight loss and anaemia.

Local complications of the colitis include toxic dilatation, severe bleeding, perforation, abscesses and strictures. The risk of developing colonic carcinoma is increased if the colitis affects the whole colon and is prolonged.

Other features include anterior uveitis, episcleritis, stomatitis, erythema nodosum, pyoderma gangrenosum, leg ulcers, arthritis, spondylitis, sacroiliitis, chronic active hepatitis, cirrhosis, pericholangitis, sclerosing cholangitis and carcinoma of the biliary tree.

The differential diagnosis of pyoderma gangrenosum includes:

1. Ulcerative colitis
2. Crohn's disease
3. Rheumatoid arthritis
4. Paraproteinaemias
5. Chronic active hepatitis
6. Lymphomas
7. Wegener's granulomatosis.

Sclerosing cholangitis affects about 3–10% of patients with ulcerative colitis (particularly those with a total colitis). It is a chronic cholestatic liver disease characterized by an obliterative inflammatory fibrosis of the biliary tract. The course of disease is variable, with most patients dying of hepatic failure. 10–30% of patients with sclerosing cholangitis will eventually develop bile duct carcinoma.

This is the CT head scan of a 70-year-old patient who has presented with a sudden onset of right-sided weakness and difficulty in speaking. He had undergone a metallic aortic valve replacement six months previously for severe aortic valve stenosis. His INR had been kept between 2 and 3 for the last six months. The clinical signs confirm that he has had a left cerebrovascular event.

What is the most appropriate management now?

1. Immediately reverse his anticoagulation with fresh frozen plasma and vitamin K
2. Continue his warfarin
3. Administer 2 mg of vitamin K and stop the warfarin only
4. Stop the warfarin only
5. Reverse his anticoagulation with fresh frozen plasma only

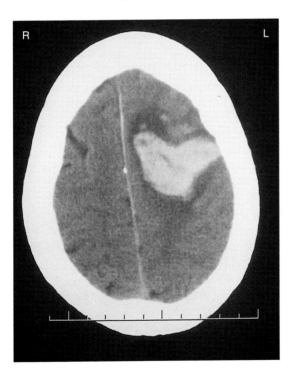

1. **Immediately reverse his anticoagulation with fresh frozen plasma and vitamin K.**

- The slide shows a large left intracerebral haematoma in the middle cerebral artery territory.
- The most appropriate management of acute haemorrhage and in this case intracranial haemorrhage in a patient receiving warfarin is to immediately reverse the anticoagulation.

For major bleeding	• Stop warfarin • Give vitamin K 5 mg slow i.v. • Give prothrombin concentrate (factors II, VII, IX, X) 50 units/kg • If there is no concentrate available then FFP (15 ml/kg).
If the INR is >8 and there is no bleeding or minor bleeding	• Stop warfarin • Give vitamin K either 0.5 mg i.v. or 5 mg p.o. Repeat dose if INR too high.
If the INR is 6.0–8.0	• Stop warfarin and remeasure the INR.

- Mechanical valves are thrombogenic and anticoagulation with a target INR of 3–4 is recommended. In the absence of atrial fibrillation anticoagulation is not required for bioprosthetic valves.
- The risk of mechanical valve embolus causing death, stroke or peripheral ischaemia requiring surgery is estimated to be 4% per year. This risk is increased with mitral valve prosthesis, ball and cage valves and multiple prosthetic valves.
- There appears to be a 7- to 10-fold increased risk of having an intracranial haemorrhage with warfarin to an absolute risk of 0.3–1.0% per year.
- The current available evidence suggests that intracranial haemorrhage occurring in patients on warfarin continues to evolve over the following 10 hours in 50% of patients.
- It seems clear therefore that anticoagulation should be reversed as soon as possible.
- There is considerable uncertainty and lack of evidence about when anticoagulation should be recommenced and a period of four to six weeks without anticoagulation has been suggested before anticoagulation should be recommenced. This needs to be balanced against the individual risk in each patient of a thromboembolic event occurring.

Question 34

This 68-year-old woman complained of gradual bilateral loss of vision, especially when reading.
  What is the most likely cause?

1. Diabetic maculopathy
2. Toxoplasmosis choroiditis
3. Age-related macular degeneration
4. Inherited central retinal dystrophy
5. Photocoagulation scarring

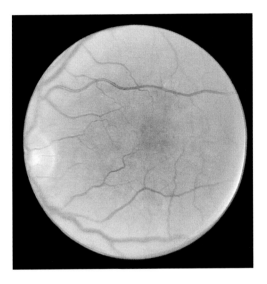

3. Age-related macular degeneration.

The most likely cause is age-related macular degeneration. There is pigmentation around the macula. This is secondary to pigment epithelial hyperplasia, which is a feature of dry, age-related macular degeneration. Other common features not present in this case include macular drusen and atrophy of the retinal pigment epithelium.

Other causes of macular pathology include diabetes, drugs such as choroquine and infections of the retina such as toxoplasma. Some patients with inherited adult-onset cerebellar ataxia or other rare neurological diseases demonstrate macular pigmentation as a feature.

What is the diagnosis in this 45-year-old woman with long-standing rheumatoid arthritis?

1. Anterior iritis
2. Scleromalacia perforans
3. Episcleritis
4. Steroid-induced scleral thinning
5. Herpetic ulcer

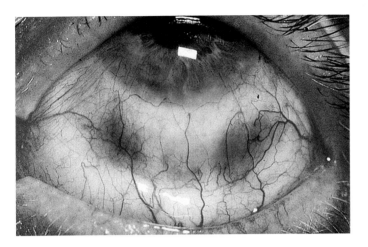

2. Scleromalacia perforans.

The slide shows the classical appearance of scleromalacia perforans, a well-recognized but rare ocular complication of rheumatoid vasculitis.

Scleritis may be classified into anterior and posterior types, and anterior scleritis may be classified into diffuse, nodular and necrotizing types. Diffuse and nodular types are usually painful and repeated attacks may lead to scleral thinning. Necrotizing scleritis is often painless and is due to the breakdown of scleral granulomas. Vision is often reduced due to the secondary complications of uveitis, keratitis, glaucoma and cataract.

Scleritis is an ophthalmological emergency requiring high-dose systemic steroids.

Ocular complications of rheumatoid arthritis include:
- Keratoconjunctivitis sicca: 25%
- Asymptomatic episcleritis
- Scleritis
- Corneal melt
- Tenosynovitis of the extraocular muscles
- Steroid-induced cataracts
- Chloroquine-associated retinopathy.

Scleritis with scleral thinning is a recognized complication of:
- Rheumatoid arthritis
- Wegener's granulomatosis
- Polyarteritis nodosa
- Ankylosing spondylitis
- Herpes zoster.

What is the clinical diagnosis?

1. Keratoderma blennorrhagicum
2. Kaposi's sarcoma
3. Tylosis
4. Tinea pedis
5. Pustular psoriasis

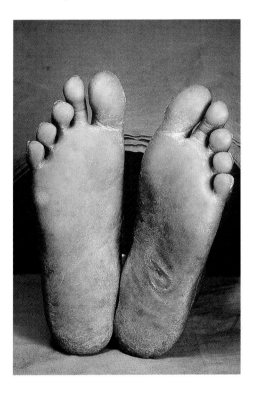

3. Tylosis.

The skin is markedly thickened and hyperkeratotic.

This is the typical appearance of tylosis or diffuse palmoplantar keratoderma.

It may be inherited as an autosomal dominant trait; in these cases the condition is usually obvious by the age of 4 years.

There is also a strong association with internal malignancy and in particular carcinoma of the oesophagus.

What is the diagnosis?

1. Papilloedema
2. Central retinal artery occlusion
3. Rubeosis iridis
4. Proliferative diabetic retinopathy
5. Central retinal vein occlusion

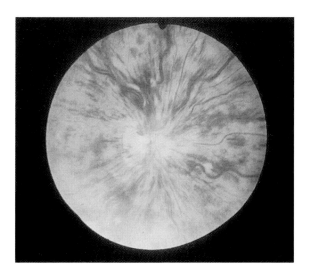

5. Central retinal vein occlusion (CRVO).

The slide shows the typical fundal changes, which include:
- Venous dilation
- Widespread haemorrhages, which may be superficial and flame-shaped or deep and blotchy
- Retinal oedema
- Cotton wool spots
- Optic disc swelling.

Causes of retinal vein occlusion:

Systemic hypertension	The retinal artery and vein share a common fascial sheath, so arteriosclerotic thickening of the artery may result in occlusion of the central retinal vein
Diabetes	
Blood dyscrasias – hyperviscosity states	Waldenström's macroglobulinaemia Polycythaemia rubra vera Less commonly, multiple myeloma
Raised intraocular pressure	Primary open-angle glaucoma

Rubeosis iridis and secondary thrombotic glaucoma are potential complications of CRVO:
- In mild cases of CRVO recanalization of the central vein may occur, with some improvement in vision.
- In severe cases retinal hypoxia stimulates neovascularization; new vessels develop primarily on the anterior surface of the iris (rubeosis iridis) approximately 90 days after the initial occlusion. Rubeosis iridis may be complicated by thrombotic glaucoma, leading to a painful blind eye which may require enucleation.

What is the ophthalmological diagnosis?

1. Toxoplasmosis choroidoretinitis
2. Grade IV hypertensive retinopathy
3. Preliferative diabetic retinopathy
4. Cytomegalovirus retinopathy
5. Candida endophthalmitis

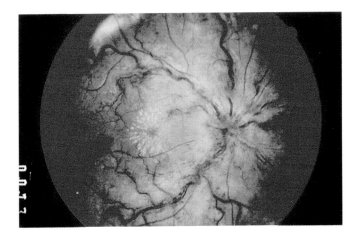

2. Grade IV hypertensive retinopathy.

The slide shows grade 4 hypertensive retinopathy due to accelerated phase hypertension. There is disc swelling, widespread haemorrhages, cotton wool spots and a macula star.

Hypertensive retinopathy may be graded:

- Grade 1: arterial constriction and heightened light reflex (copper/silver wiring)
- Grade 2: arterial venous nipping
- Grade 3: haemorrhages, cotton wool spots and hard exudates (macula star)
- Grade 4: consists of all the grade 3 changes in addition to silver wiring of arterioles and disc swelling.

This is a coeliac axis angiogram of a 49-year-old male who presented with a one-year history of fever and a flitting arthralgia. He was recently being investigated for weakness in his right hand. On this occasion he has presented with severe abdominal pain.

What is the diagnosis?

1. Polyarteritis nodosa
2. Henoch–Schönlein purpura
3. Wegener's granulomatosis
4. Syphilis
5. Giant cell arteritis

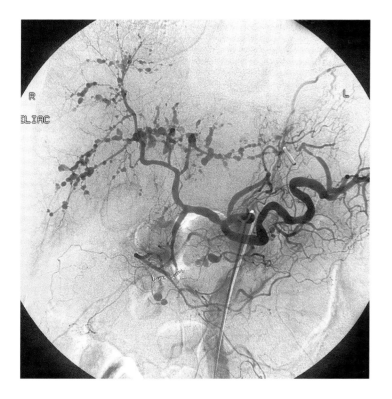

1. Polyarteritis nodosa.

The angiogram shows the classical features of polyarteritis nodosa.

Polyarteritis nodosa is a vasculitis of medium-sized arteries in which aneurysm formation is a frequent occurrence.

Typically a patient is middle-aged and males are more commonly affected. They tend to present with fever, weight loss and night sweats. The hand weakness suggests that he may have developed a mononeuritis multiplex, which is a recognized complication.

Abdominal pain secondary to intestinal ischaemia is a common symptom.

There are no specific diagnostic features. Anti-neutrophil cytoplasmic antibodies are usually negative. Angiographic studies will reveal evidence of vasculitis in muscular arteries with aneurysmal formation.

Patients respond well to immunosuppressive treatment regimens with prednisolone and cyclophosphamide.

This male presented aged 12 with a haemolytic anaemia. What is the diagnosis?

1. Systemic lupus erythematosus
2. Refsum's disease
3. Ehlers–Danlos syndrome
4. Haemochromatosis
5. Wilson's disease

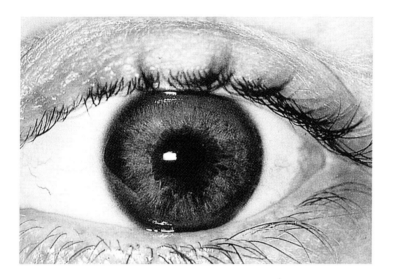

5. Wilson's disease.

The slide shows a Kayser–Fleischer ring. The typical golden appearance of copper deposition in the limbus of the cornea is shown.

The most likely underlying diagnosis is Wilson's disease, which may present with a Coombs-negative haemolytic anaemia in 10% of cases.

Wilson's disease is an autosomal recessive disorder due to mutation of a gene on the long arm of chromosome 13. It is characterized by absent or greatly reduced caeruloplasmin plasma levels but the pathogenetic abnormality is a reduction in the biliary excretion of copper. Tissue levels of copper are high, especially in the liver, brain, cornea and kidney.

Clinical features include:

1. Haematological: Coombs-negative haemolysis 10%
2. Hepatic: 50% will present with liver derangement
   — Hepatitis
   — Cirrhosis with portal hypertension; rarely may present with fulminant hepatic failure
   — Pigment gallstones due to haemolysis
3. Neurological
   — Behavioural problems
   — Parkinsonian features and chorea
4. Renal: proximal renal tubular acidosis
5. Ocular: Kayser–Fleischer ring
6. Musculoskeletal: early osteoarthritis
7. Nails: blue nails.

The diagnosis is confirmed by the demonstration of either:
- A serum ceruloplasmin level <20 mg/dL *and* Kayser–Fleischer rings or
- A serum ceruloplasmin level <20 mg/dL *and* a concentration of copper in a liver biopsy sample >250 µg/g dry weight.
- 24-hour copper urine collections will always be raised in Wilson's disease but can also occur in other liver diseases.

Treatment includes a low-copper diet, copper chelation with penicillamine, trientine or oral zinc (may prevent copper absorption). In cases where the presentation is of fulminant hepatic failure, a liver transplant will be required.

This is the peripheral blood film from an asymptomatic 35-year-old man in whom a raised white cell count was found during a routine medical check-up. Examination of his abdomen revealed 6 cm splenomegaly.

What is the likely diagnosis?

1. Acute myeloid leukaemia
2. Acute lymphoblastic leukaemia
3. Chronic myeloid leukaemia
4. Myelofibrosis
5. Chronic lymphatic leukaemia

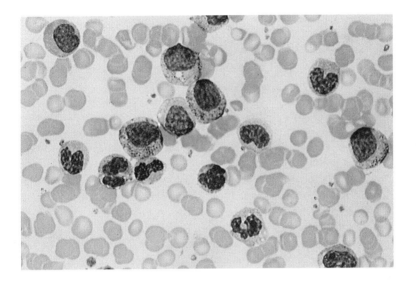

3. Chronic myeloid leukaemia.

The blood film shows an increased number of neutrophils, one myelocyte and a basophil.

These are consistent with a diagnosis of chronic myeloid leukaemia (CML).

Finding the Philadelphia chromosome in blood or bone marrow would confirm the diagnosis.

An increased neutrophil count coupled with the presence of immature myeloid precursors and basophilia in the peripheral blood is a typical presentation of CML.

Basophilia is a feature of myeloproliferative disorders in general and may be striking in CML.

Leukaemoid reactions: where there is a marked leukocytosis (usually greater than $50\ 000 \times 10^9$ L) and immature myeloid precursors circulate in the peripheral blood, can be seen associated with sepsis, carcinoma of the lung or stomach, Hodgkin's disease or dermatitis herpetiformis. Very occasionally the blood film may be difficult to differentiate from that seen in CML. However, in a leukaemoid reaction the neutrophils usually show toxic granulation and Döhle bodies, which are absent in CML, and the karyotype in a leukaemoid reaction is normal.

Other useful laboratory indicators in favour of a diagnosis of CML are a low neutrophil alkaline phosphatase, raised serum urate, and an elevated level of vitamin B_{12} and its binding protein transcobalamin. The Philadelphia chromosome is formed by a reciprocal translocation of the distal part of the long arms of chromosomes 9 and 22. This causes the abl gene, normally present on chromosome 9, to move to a position adjacent to the bcr gene on chromosome 22, resulting in the formation of a novel bcrabl gene. This new gene codes for a 210 kDa protein with tyrosine kinase activity which is likely to be involved in the pathogenesis of CML. Imatimib is a protein tyrosine kinase inhibitor that is licensed for the treatment of CML.

Note: A Philadelphia chromosome is occasionally found in acute lymphoblastic leukaemia, where it codes for a similar but smaller protein.

Question 42

This man presented with diplopia and has recently been investigated by cardiologists for syncopal episodes.

What is the likely underlying diagnosis?

1. Retinitis pigmentosa
2. Kearns–Sayre syndrome
3. Friedreich's ataxia
4. Duchenne muscular dystrophy
5. Graves' disease

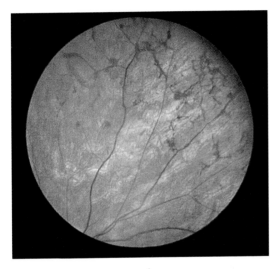

2. Kearns–Sayre syndrome.

The slide shows the typical appearance of retinitis pigmentosa. There is scattering of black pigment, which has a 'bone spicule' appearance.

The Kearns–Sayre syndrome can be considered a triad of:

1. Retinitis pigmentosa
2. Progressive external ophthalmoplegia
3. Cardiac conduction defects.

It presents before the age of 20 years.

Other findings include ataxia, an elevated CSF protein, deafness, short stature, diabetes and hypoparathyroidism.

Deletions of mitochondrial DNA in muscle biopsies are seen in over 80% of such patients.

Retinitis pigmentosa can be inherited as an isolated disorder or in association with a number of systemic conditions that include:

- Laurence–Moon–Biedl–Bardet syndrome
- Abetalipoproteinaemia
- Refsum's disease
- Kearns–Sayre syndrome
- Usher's syndrome
- Autosomal dominant cerebellar ataxia syndromes.

a What are the changes on this slide consistent with?
   1. Pre-proliferative diabetic retinopathy
   2. Proliferative diabetic retinopathy
   3. Diabetic maculopathy
   4. Rubeosis iridis
   5. Background retinopathy

b What treatment would be the most appropriate management step for this patient?
   1. Commence an ACEI
   2. Focal photocoagulation
   3. Immediate ophthalmological referral
   4. Tight glycaemic control
   5. Yearly ophthalmological screening

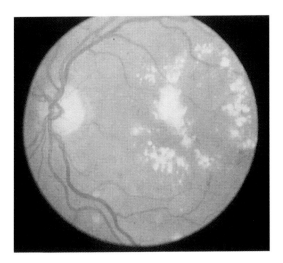

a 3. Diabetic maculopathy
b 2. Focal photocoagulation.

Diabetic eye disease is the commonest cause of blindness in the United Kingdom between the ages of 20 and 65 years. Diabetic retinopathy is present in approximately 25% of cases of juvenile-onset insulin-dependent diabetes after 10 years and approximately 50% of adult non-insulin-dependent diabetic patients after 10 years.

Classification of diabetic eye disease

Background	Visual acuity is unaffected. *Microaneurysms*: outpouchings of the capillary wall appear as small round dots temporal to the macula. *Dot and blot haemorrhages*: represent leakage of fluid and microproteins; they originate from the venous end of capillaries and flame-shaped haemorrhages originating from the superficial arterioles. *Hard exudates*: have a yellow waxy appearance. *Retinal oedema*: can only be seen with a slit-lamp examination.
Diabetic maculopathy	*Oedema, exudates* and *ischaemia* affecting the macula. Central vision is lost; peripheral vision is maintained.
Preproliferative retinopathy	*Cotton wool spots* (hold-up of axonoplasmic flow, evidence of microvascular ischaemia).
Proliferative retinopathy	*Neovascularization* (develops in response to ischaemia). The new vessels are liable to haemorrhage into the vitreous, with subsequent fibrosis, retinal detachment and loss of vision.
Rubeosis iridis	*New vessel formation* on the surface of the iris, may be complicated by glaucoma.
Cataracts	*Snowflake cataract* of poorly controlled juvenile diabetes.

- Patients with type I diabetes are more likely to develop proliferative disease than maculopathy, whereas patients with type II disease are more likely to develop a maculopathy.

Treatment of diabetic eye disease
- Maculopathy due to hard exudate deposits can be successfully treated if caught early by focal photocoagulation of the leaking vessels adjacent to the macula.
- All patients with diabetes mellitus will have a significant improvement in microvascular and macrovascular end-points with tight glycaemic control.
- Neovascularization of the retina is an indication for argon laser panretinal photocoagulation.

This 40-year-old woman presented with a two-year history of malaise and arthralgia affecting the small joints of the hands. Investigations have shown a persistently elevated ESR of 30–50 mm in the first hour. She then complained of a dull ache in her left forearm while ironing.

What is the diagnosis?

1. Polyarteritis nodosa
2. Giant cell arteritis
3. Takayasu arteritis
4. Syphilitic aortitis
5. Kawasaki's disease

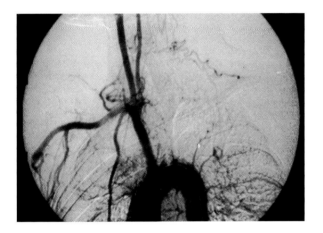

3. Takayasu arteritis.

The picture shows a digital subtraction arch aortogram that shows occlusion of the left common carotid and left subclavian arteries.

Takayasu arteritis is a large-vessel vasculitis affecting predominantly the aortic arch and its proximal branches.

- It classically presents in young women of <40 years with systemic symptoms of fever, malaise, arthralgia, weight loss and upper limb claudication.
- On clinical examination unequal limb pulses are typical, with hypertension a prominent feature, reflecting renal vessel involvement. Examination of the eyes may reveal retinal haemorrhages, AV fistulae and atrophy of the iris. Aortic regurgitation may be present.
- The ESR and CRP are usually raised. Angiography is the gold standard investigation.
- Immunosuppressive treatment with corticosteroids, cyclophosphamide and azathioprine have improved the prognosis.

The differential diagnosis of unequal limb pulses includes:
- Takayasu's arteritis
- Giant cell arteritis
- Syphilitic aortitis
- Aortic dissection
- Thrombosis and emboli
- Buerger's disease
- Abnormal vessel development.

Note:
- Polyarteritis nodosa is a medium-vessel vasculitis characterized by micro-aneurysm formation along branches of the coeliac axis and renal arteries.
- Kawasaki disease is a medium vasculitis of childhood characterized by involvement of the coronary arteries.
- Giant cell arteritis is a disease of the elderly and does not occur in patients less than 50 years of age. It affects the aorta and its major branches, with a predilection for the extracranial branches of the carotid artery.
- Syphilis is a well-recognized cause of aortitis with aneurysm formation, affecting particularly the ascending aorta, leading to aortic incompetence and possible rupture.

This 17-year-old South American girl presented with the lesion shown below.

The chemotherapeutic agent of choice is:

1. Diethylcarbamazine
2. i.v. amphotericin
3. Tiabendazole
4. Praziquantel
5. Sodium stibogluconate

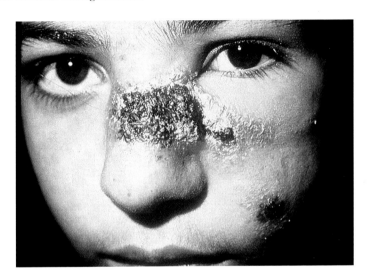

5. **Sodium stibogluconate.**

The slide shows the typical appearance of **cutaneous leishmaniasis**. This is caused by parasites of the genus *Leishmania*; at least 12 species cause disease in man. *Leishmania brasiliensis brasiliensis* is the major cause of American cutaneous leishmaniasis. The vector is the sand-fly; forest rodents are the likely reservoir of infection.

Leishmania inoculated into the skin by the sand-fly bite multiply in macrophages and cause a nodule which increases in size over several weeks. The crust often falls off, leaving a painless ulcer, which eventually heals leaving a disfiguring scar.

Approximately 40% of patients with cutaneous ulcers due to *L. brasiliensis brasiliensis* infection will develop mucocutaneous leishmaniasis (espundia) with involvement of the nasal mucosa, pharynx, palate and lip. Untreated mucocutaneous leishmaniasis tends to progress slowly, eventually destroying the nose and face.

Diagnosis can be confirmed by detecting the parasites in material obtained from a lesion; the material is smeared, stained (Giemsa stain) and examined for intracellular parasites. Material is also inoculated into specific culture media or into hamsters.

The *Leishmania* skin test is positive in approximately 90% of cases of cutaneous and mucocutaneous leishmaniasis.

Systemic treatment of *L. brasiliensis brasiliensis* with pentavalent antimonials, e.g. sodium stibogluconate, is effective and prevents the disfiguring espundia from developing.

This patient has noticed right-sided clumsiness and has been choking on her food. She has also noticed numbness of her face on the same side. The GP has also made the referral, however, because she has noticed pain in her left leg and the concern is that she may have developed left deep vein thrombosis.

What vascular territory may account for all her clinical features?

1. Middle and anterior cerebral artery territory
2. Posterior and middle cerebral artery territory
3. Anterior cerebral artery territory
4. Posterior inferior cerebellar artery
5. Lacunar territory

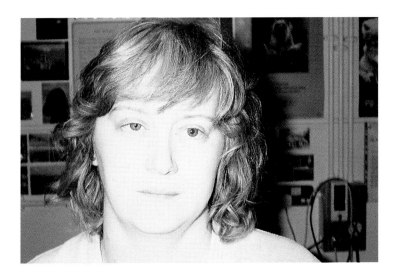

4. Posterior inferior cerebellar artery.

The slide shows that the patient has a right Horner's syndrome.
She has an ipsilateral ptosis and a meiosis (smaller pupil).
  Associated features can also include:

- Enophthalmos
- Impaired sweating over the forehead
- A blocked nose, and a bloodshot cornea.

Horner's syndrome and the other clinical features can be accounted for by occlusion of the posterior inferior cerebellar artery. This constellation of features is called the lateral medullary syndrome (*Wallenberg's syndrome*).
  The patient would be expected to have:

- An ipsilateral Horner's syndrome (descending sympathetic tract)
- Ipsilateral cerebellar signs (cerebellum and its connections), palatal paralysis (dysphagia and hoarseness due to a vocal cord paralysis – IXth and Xth nerves)
- Ipsilateral decreased trigeminal pain and temperature sensation (descending tract and nucleus of the Vth nerve)
- The patient may also have contralateral pain and temperature loss in the limbs due to involvement of the spinothalamic tract
- Vestibular involvement may produce nystagmus, diplopia, nausea and vomiting.

Horner's syndrome results from any lesion interrupting the sympathetic supply to the eye.
  There are three neurones involved:

- The first passes from the hypothalamus to the lateral grey matter in the thoracic cord.
- The second passes from the cord, via the T1 root, to the superior cervical ganglion.
- The third, from the superior cervical ganglion, follows the carotid artery to join the long ciliary and third cranial nerves to supply the pupil and levator palpebrae superioris.

Causes of Horner's syndrome include:

- Hypothalamic lesions
- Brain stem lesions, e.g. lateral medullary syndrome
- Cervical cord lesions, e.g. syringomyelia
- Lesions affecting T1 spinal root, e.g. Pancoast tumour
- Lesions affecting the sympathetic chain, e.g. surgery, trauma, neoplasm.

What is the clinical diagnosis?

1. Cutaneous larva migrans
2. Scabies
3. Cutaneous leishmaniasis
4. Tuberculoid leprosy
5. Erythema gyratum repens

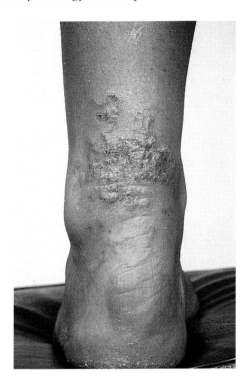

1. Cutaneous larva migrans.

This is the typical appearance of larva migrans: the migration of larvae under the skin accompanied by urticarial wheals. Causes include:

1. *Ancylostoma braziliense* and *A. caninum* (hookworms): intestinal parasites of dogs which cause larva migrans in man. The larvae progress irregularly at 1 cm/hour. The advancing end of the burrow is red and itchy, the older part brown and scaly. Treatment is by local application of tiabendazole.
2. *Strongyloides stercoralis* (a nematode) endemic in the tropics, especially the Far East. Man is the chief natural host. Clinical features include local itch at the initial site of larval entry, typical linear urticarial wheals (these may extend at the rate of 3 cm per hour and are hence referred to as 'larva currens', symptoms attributable to gut infestation, e.g. anaemia, diarrhoea, malabsorption, ileus and volvulus, heavy infection that may be associated with asthma or alveolar haemorrhage. *Strongyloides* is best treated with oral tiabendazole or ivermectin.

Drug treatment for some protozoal and helminthic infections

Leishmaniasis	Sodium stibogluconate
Trypanosomiasis	Suramine, melarosopol
Toxoplasmosis	Pyrimethamine and sulfadiazine
Toxocara	Diethylcarbamazine/albendazole
Threadworms (*Enteromoebius vermicularis*)	Mebendazole/piperazine
Roundworms (*Ascaris lumbricoides*)	Levamisole/mebendazole/piperazine
Tapeworms, e.g. cysticercosis	Niclosamide/praziquantel
Hyatid (*Echinococcus granulosus*)	Albendazole
Hookworm (*Ancylostoma duodenale*)	Mebendazole
Schistosomiasis	Praziquantel
Filarial infections	Diethylcarbamazine, ivermectin
Cutaneous larva migrans	Tiabendazole/albendazole
Strongyloides	Tiabendazole, ivermectin
Pneumocystis carinii	Co-trimoxazole Atorvaquone Pentamidine Clindamycin and primiquine

a What treatment would you initiate?
1. Nifedipine
2. Nimodipine
3. Dexamethasone
4. i.v. broad-spectrum antibiotics
5. Aspirin

b What is the next investigation that you would organize?
1. Lumbar puncture
2. MRI brain
3. Digital subtraction angiography
4. Erythrocyte sedimentation rate
5. Chest X ray

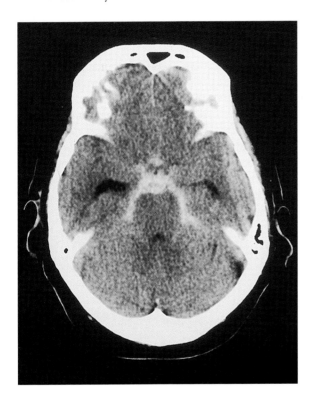

a 2. Nimodipine
b 3. Digital subtraction angiography.

The CT image shows high-attenuation material consistent with blood in the ventricles; this is consistent with a diagnosis of subarachnoid haemorrhage.

- A high-resolution CT head scan is the first investigation of choice. Where there is a history suggestive of subarachnoid haemorrhage it should be carried out as an emergency investigation.
- With a convincing history but a negative scan a lumber puncture should be taken 6–12 hours after the onset of headache and sent for xanthochromic analysis.
- Subsequent investigations are aimed at discovering the aneurysmal source. Digital subtraction angiography is the gold standard. CT and MRI angiography are rapidly evolving non-invasive techniques that are being used with increasing frequency.

Nimodipine is at present the only pharmacological agent that has shown any clinical benefit by reducing the frequency of cerebral ischaemia, thereby reducing cerebral infarction and improving outcome. It is a cerebral calcium antagonist but the exact mechanism of neuroprotection is unclear.

An oral dose of 60 mg 4-hourly is given. If the patient is comatosed, intravenous nimodipine can be administered provided hypotension has been corrected. Surgery may be required in the acute resuscitation process if there is evidence of raised intracranial pressure, requiring the insertion of an external ventricular drain.

This 60-year-old smoker complained of persistent cough and difficulty in climbing stairs.

Which of the following would not be consistent with the underlying diagnosis?

1. A heliotrope rash
2. Anti-Mi-2 antibody
3. A normal CK level
4. An association with underlying bronchial carcinoma
5. Large-amplitude and long-duration polyphasic motor unit potentials

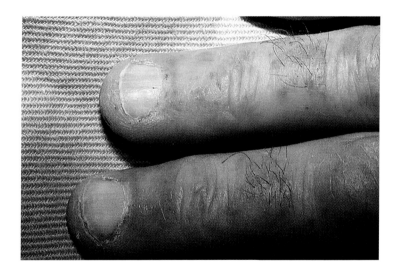

5. Large-amplitude and long-duration polyphasic motor unit potentials.

The purple plaques over the knuckles are Gottron's papules and these are a well-recognized cutaneous manifestation of dermatomyositis. The characteristic neurophysiological changes seen with dermatositis and polymyositis are polyphasic motor potentials of a short duration and low amplitude. In contrast, large-amplitude and long-duration polyphasic motor unit potentials are seen with neuropathic disorders.

Dermatomyositis, or polymyositis without the rash, are the commonest forms of idiopathic inflammatory myopathies. Proximal muscle weakness is the additional dominating clinical feature. An underlying malignancy is present in up to 15% of patients over the age of 45 and they should therefore be investigated accordingly. The history of persistent cough in a smoker suggests the possibility of an underlying bronchial carcinoma.

Other cutaneous manifestations of dermatomyositis include:

- A heliotropic rash on the eyelids, cheeks and light exposed areas
- Nail-fold changes with periungual erythema, cuticular hypertrophy and infarcts
- Sclerodermatous skin changes with cutaneous and muscular calcification.

A diagnosis of dermatomyositis requires three of the following four criteria to be present in addition to the characteristic rash:

1. Proximal muscle weakness – usually symmetrical
2. Elevated serum levels of muscle enzymes
3. Typical muscle biopsy changes
4. The triad of electromyographic changes: polyphasic, short, small motor unit potentials; high-frequency repetitive discharges; and spontaneous fibrillation.

Serology in dermatositis:

- 40–80% of patients with PM and DM are ANA positive.
- Anti-Mi-2 antibodies are seen in up to 10% of patients with classical dermatomyositis and are associated with a good prognosis.
- The antisynthetase antibodies anti Jo-1, PL-7 and PL-12 are seen in the antisynthetase syndrome; the main features are: polymyositis > dermatomyositis, interstitial lung disease in 50%, non-erosive arthritis and mechanic's hands.
- Anti-SRP is associated with acute-onset severe polymyositis with cardiac involvement and a poor prognosis

Note: Amyotrophic dermatomyositis is well recognized. In these cases the cutaneous manifestations of DM occur in the absence of clinically apparent muscle involvement. Over time approximately 50% of patients will show muscle involvement but a significant proportion will manifest skin disease only. Patients can therefore present with dermatomyositis but have *normal* creatinine kinase levels.

This 54-year-old smoker presented with weakness and loss of sensation in his left hand. Further investigation revealed him to have a right bronchogenic carcinoma.

What is the likely diagnosis?

1. Pancoast's syndrome
2. Left ulnar nerve lesion
3. Left radial nerve palsy
4. Left carpal tunnel syndrome
5. Dupuytren's contracture

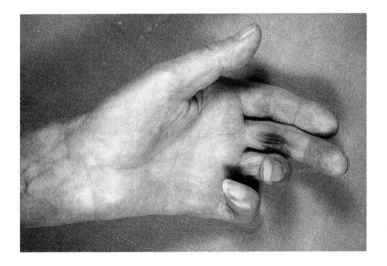

2. Left ulnar nerve lesion.

This slide shows the typical features of a left claw hand secondary to an ulnar nerve palsy. There is wasting of the small hand muscles, with preservation of the thenar eminence. This would be typical of an ulnar nerve palsy.

This may be isolated or part of a mononeuritis multiplex picture secondary to right-sided bronchial carcinoma.

Clawing is due to hyperextension at the MCP joint and flexion of the IP joint. Clawing is more pronounced with an ulnar nerve lesion at the wrist. A lesion at or above the elbow also causes loss of digitorum profundus and therefore less flexion at the interphalangeal joints. The clawing is only seen in the fourth and fifth fingers because the median nerve supplies the radial or (lateral) two lumbricals.

Examination would reveal:

- Wasting of the hypothenar eminence
- Sensory loss over the fifth finger and adjacent half of the fourth finger, in addition to medial and palmer aspects of the hand.
- Weakness of all small hand muscles except: The lateral two lumbricals, opponens pollicis brevis, abductor pollicis brevis, and flexor pollicis longus (**loaf**): these are supplied by the median nerve.

The causes of a mononeuritis multiplex include:

- Diabetes
- Malignancy
- Sarcoid
- Churg–Strauss syndrome
- Rheumatoid arthritis
- Tuberculous leprosy
- Lyme disease.

Note:

- A Pancoast syndrome refers to a lower brachial plexus damage due to local invasion by an apical tumour. This will give weakness in the C8, T1, T2 distribution (i.e. of all the hand muscles). If there is involvement of the cervical sympathetic trunk there may also be an associated Horner's syndrome. (The bronchogenic carcinoma in this case is on the opposite side to the hand weakness.)
- A T1 root lesion will cause weakness and wasting of *all* the intrinsic hand muscles.

a Which organism is responsible for this?
  1. Onchocerciasis
  2. *Loa loa*
  3. *Wuchereria bancrofti*
  4. Larva currens
  5. Dracunculosis

b Which of the following treatments would you use?
  1. Praziquantel
  2. Sodium stibogluconate
  3. Melarosopol
  4. Diethylcarbamazine
  5. Tiabendazole

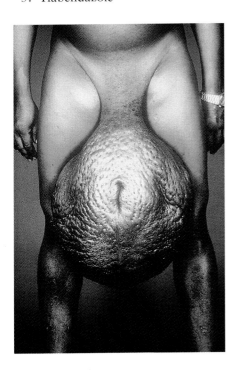

a 3. *Wuchereria bancrofti*
b 4. Diethylcarbamazine.

This is the typical appearance of lymphatic filariasis and has led to elephantiasis of the scrotum in this case.

Three species of lymphatic dwelling filarial worms – *Wuchereria bancrofti*, *Brugia malayi* and *B. timori* – cause lymphatic filariasis in humans. The vectors are species of mosquitoes. The most significant complication of these infections is lymphatic filariasis causing lymphoedema, elephantiasis and hydroceles. *Bancrofti* filariasis commonly affects the male genitals with hydrocele formation and elephantiasis usually takes the form of unilateral involvement of the whole lower limb. Brugian filariasis never involves the genitals and elephantiasis is restricted to the arm below the elbow or the leg below the knee.

All filarial infections can present with a spectrum of disease:
- No manifestations
- Asymptomatic microfilaemia
- Filarial fever
- Chronic lymphatic pathology
- Tropical pulmonary eosinophilia.

The treatment of choice for filarial infections is diethylcarbamazine.

(*W. bancrofti* is distributed throughout the tropical regions of Asia, Africa, the Americas and the Pacific. *B. malayi* is found in South East Asia. *B. timori* occurs only on some small islands in Indonesia.)

What is the ophthalmological diagnosis?

1. Optic disc cupping
2. Papilloedema
3. Angioid streaks
4. Optic atrophy
5. Optic disc drusen

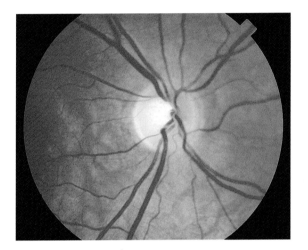

4. Optic atrophy.

The slide shows the classical appearance of optic atrophy, with a very pale, well-demarcated disc.

Causes of optic atrophy are as follows:

Hereditary causes

- *Leber's optic atrophy*: transmitted on mitochondrial DNA, commoner in males, uniocular visual loss in the second or third decade which eventually becomes bilateral.
- *Friedreich's ataxia*: autosomal recessive, occasionally autosomal dominant. Symptoms classically present between the ages of 8 and 16 years. The disease is slowly progressive and few patients live for more than 20 years after onset of the disease.
  Clinical features:
  — High arched palate/kyphoscoliosis/bilateral pes cavus
  — Cerebellar signs: ataxia, dysarthria, nystagmus
  — Dorsal column loss: impaired vibration and position sense
  — Peripheral neuropathy
  — Optic atrophy
  — Corticospinal tract involvement: extensor plantar responses
  — Cardiomyopathy
  — Diabetes.
- *DIDMOAD syndrome*: diabetes insipidus, diabetes mellitus, optic atrophy and deafness.
- *Retinitis pigmentosa*.

Acquired causes

- Ischaemia: temporal arteritis, retinal artery occlusion
- Demyelination
- Infections: choroidoretinitis
- Metabolic causes: vitamin B_{12} deficiency, diabetes mellitus
- Toxic causes: lead, methyl alcohol, tobacco/alcohol ambylopia, cyanide
- Chronic papilloedema
- Glaucoma
- Paget's disease
- Trauma leading to nerve section
- Tumours compressing the optic nerve.

a What is the commonest lesion to cause this appearance?
   1. Lymphoma
   2. Aneurysm of the basilar artery
   3. Cholesteatoma
   4. Meningioma
   5. Acoustic neuroma

b Which clinical sign is *least* likely as a result of this lesion?
   1. Unilateral deafness
   2. Unilateral absent corneal reflex
   3. Right VIIth nerve palsy
   4. Numbness in ophthalmic division of the trigeminal nerve
   5. Canal paresis on vestibular testing

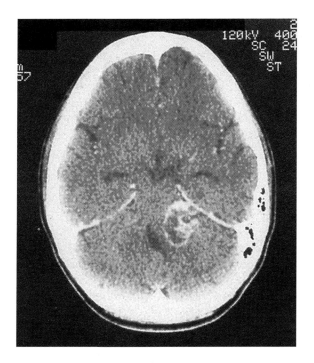

a 5. Acoustic neuroma
b 3. Right VIIth nerve palsy.

The CT scan shows a right cerebellopontine angle-enhancing lesion.
    Acoustic neuromas are the commonest lesions occurring in the cerebellopontine angle.
    Other causes of cerebellopontine angle lesions include:

1. Meningioma
2. Cholesteatoma
3. Haemangioblastoma
4. Neuromas affecting the Vth, VIIth and Xth cranial nerves
5. Aneurysm of the basilar artery
6. Medulloblastoma
7. Lymphomatous deposits
8. Nasopharyngeal carcinoma.

- The cerebellopontine angle (triangle) comprises the cerebellum, lateral pons and inner third of the petrous bone. Lesions affect the Vth, VIth, VIIth, VIIIth and IXth cranial nerves.
- Acoustic neuromas arise from the vestibular division of the VIIIth cranial nerve, and commonly present in the fourth and fifth decades.
- The tumours are usually well encapsulated and unilateral; bilateral lesions occur, particularly in association with Von Recklinghausen's disease.
- The effects of pressure on the immediate structures around the neuroma predominate; raised intracranial pressure is a late feature. Tinnitus and deafness are the earliest symptoms, followed by vertigo. Loss of the corneal reflex, as the trigeminal nerve is lifted up by the neuroma, is usually the earliest sign detected, followed by numbness in the distribution of the Vth nerve. Other signs include decreased auditory acuity, canal paresis on vestibular testing, and later paresis of the VIth (leading to a convergent strabismus), VIIth, and IXth nerves (although the VIIth nerve is remarkably resilient to compression).
- Late manifestations include ipsilateral cerebellar signs and brain stem compression.

Note: Canal paresis is where the semicircular canals in the inner ear fail to respond to caloric testing.

This 14-year-old boy presented to casualty with sudden-onset weakness of the right arm and leg. His peripheral blood film is shown.
The likely diagnosis is:

1. Homocystinuria
2. Sickle cell disease
3. Abetalipoproteinaemia
4. Thrombotic thrombocytopenia
5. Antiphospholipid antibody syndrome

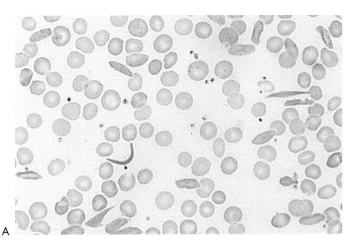

A

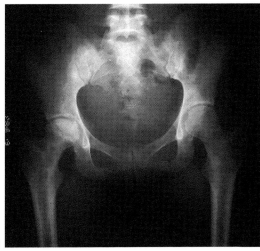

B

2. Sickle cell disease.

The peripheral blood film shows irreversibly sickled cells (crescenteric cells with two pointed extremities). Other features that may be seen on the blood film include target cells (although these are not as prominent as in HbSC disease) and Howell–Jolly bodies caused by splenic infarction and consequent asplenism. The X-ray shows avascular necrosis of the right femoral head.

Sickle cell anaemia arises due to a substitution of valine for glutamic acid at position 6 of the beta chain. HbS (Hb alpha-2, beta-S2) is insoluble and forms crystals when exposed to low oxygen tensions. This causes red cells to sickle, leading to tissue and organ infarction.

Clinical features of sickle cell anaemia:

- A *severe haemolytic anaemia* punctuated by *crises*. The clinical expression is variable, with some patients having very mild disease, while others have severe disease with many crises.
- Crises:
  — *Painful vascular occlusive crises*: precipitated by hypoxia, acidosis, infection, dehydration or acidosis. Infarcts can occur in a variety of organs: bones, spleen, lungs and brain or spinal cord. Stroke may occur in up to 7% of patients. The hand–foot syndrome occurs in children: infarcts of the small bones leading to painful dactylitis and digits of varying length.
  — *Visceral sequestration crises*: due to sickling within organs, e.g. liver, bones, leading to severe anaemia. A severe chest syndrome with infiltrates on the chest X-ray is the commonest cause of death.
  — *Aplastic crises*: secondary to parvovirus infection or folate deficiency. Leads to a sudden drop in Hb with a low reticulocyte count.
  — *Haemolytic crises*: an increased rate of haemolysis, leading to a fall in haemoglobin but a rise in the reticulocyte count.
- Other clinical features include: leg ulcers, splenomegaly in early childhood, hyposplenism due to autoinfarction in adolescents, proliferative retinopathy, priapism, pigment gallstones, abnormal liver function tests secondary to microinfarcts, renal papillary necrosis, nephrogenic diabetes insipidus and occasionally glomerulosclerosis.

Treatment

- *General measures*: daily folic acid supplements, pneumococcal vaccination, regular oral penicillin: avoid factors known to precipitate crises.
- *Management of crises*: analgesics, treat underlying infection if present, ensure adequate oxygenation (15% require intubation), rehydration, blood transfusion for severe anaemia, exchange transfusion for neurological damage or sequestration crisis.

Other notes: Sickle cell disease: haemoglobin electrophoresis will show HbS, HbF and HbA2 but not HbA. In contrast with sickle cell trait a relatively benign condition with no anaemia and normal appearance of red cells on the film but crises can be caused by extreme anoxic or infectious stresses where haemoglobin electrophoresis will show HbS (25–40% of total Hb), HbF, HbA and HBA2.

The most likely diagnosis in this 80-year-old is:

1. Osteoarthritis
2. Arterial ulcer
3. Tophaceous gout
4. Staphylococcal ulcer
5. Eroded rheumatoid nodule

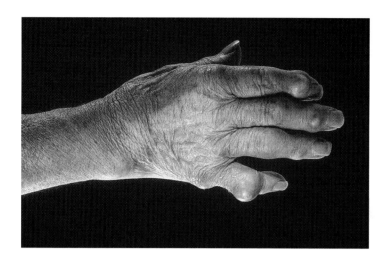

3. Tophaceous gout.

This slide shows the typical appearances of chronic tophaceous gout.

Gout progresses from hyperuricaemia to regular attacks of acute gout and, if left untreated, after a decade to chronic tophaceous gout. This stage is characterized by:

1. Tophi: chalky deposits containing urate crystals which may occur anywhere but are most commonly found on the ears, hands, around affected joints and occasionally in bursae.
2. Gouty joint erosions which are juxta-articular and generally large.

The rate of formation of tophi is a function of the degree and duration of the hyperuricaemia. As tophi and urate-induced renal disease advance, acute attacks of gout occur less frequently. The tophi themselves are not painful but do cause a crippling deformity. Complications of the tophi include ulceration, infection and rarely bony ankylosis. Tophi may occur in the myocardium, mitral valve, cardiac conduction system, eye and larynx, and may even cause spinal compression.

- Colchicine is an alkaloid that rapidly relieves the pain and inflammation of an acute attack.
- NSAIDs (but not aspirin, which causes urate retention) are also effective treatments for acute gout.
- Allopurinol is an xanthine oxidase inhibitor. This is the enzyme that converts xanthine and hypoxanthine to uric acid. Allopurinol therapy will lower uric acid levels and can prevent recurrent acute attacks of gout. Allopurinol therapy should not be started during an acute attack and when patients are commenced on treatment colchicine or an NSAID should be co-prescribed for the first two–four weeks to prevent acute attacks during this period.

Note: Gouty tophi may also occur in patients who have never experienced an acute attack of gout: typically elderly patients with heart failure treated with furosemide (frusemide).

What is the haematological diagnosis?

1. Myelofibrosis
2. Microangiopathic haemolytic anaemia
3. Acanthocytosis
4. Elliptocytosis
5. Thalassaemia major

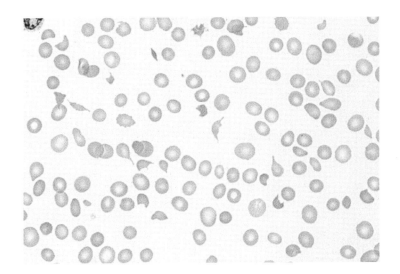

2. Microangiopathic haemolytic anaemia.

The slide shows the classical appearance of a microangiopathic haemolytic anaemia (MAHA) with helmet cells, red cell fragments and a number of contracted and deeply staining cells. There is also a paucity of platelets in the slide.

MAHA describes intravascular haemolysis with fragmentation of red cells caused by their destruction in an abnormal microcirculation. The blood film characteristically shows microspherocytes and fragmented red cells (helmet cells).

Three main pathological processes lead to MAHA:
- The deposition of fibrin strands such as occurs in disseminated intravascular coagulation (DIC).
- Platelet adherence and aggregation – thrombotic microangiopathies TTP and HUS.
- Vasculitis as caused by autoimmune disorders and sepsis.

Causes of MAHA:

Thrombotic microangiopathies	Thrombotic thombocytopenic purpura (TTP) Haemolytic uraemic syndrome (HUS)
Accelerated hypertension	
Acute glomerular nephritis	
Pre-eclampsia HELLP	(haemolysis, elevated liver enzymes, low platelets)
Vasculitides	Polyarteritis nodosa Wegener's granulomatosis SLE
Drugs	Mitomycin C, ciclosporin
Malignancy	
Septicaemia	
Primary pulmonary hypertension	
Cavernous haemangioma	
(Prosthetic valve-induced haemolysis)	A mechanical haemolysis

Remember that:
- The platelet count will be normal in a pure MAHA.
- The platelet count will be low but the PT, aPTT and fibrinogen normal in the thrombotic thromboangiopathies: HUS and TTP.
- The platelet count will be low, PT and APTT prolonged, fibrinogen low and fibrin degradation products raised in DIC.

This is the blood film of a 27-year-old patient who presented with a fever. The chest X-ray showed widespread shadowing.

What is the *least* likely clinical diagnosis?

1. Microscopic polyarteritis
2. *Strongyloides stercoralis*
3. *Aspergillus fumigatus*
4. Tetracycline use
5. Churg–Strauss syndrome

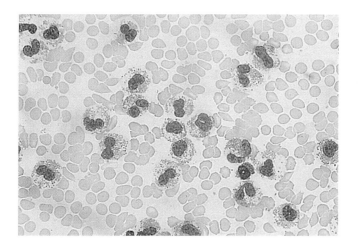

1. Microscopic polyarteritis.

The blood film shows an increased number of eosinophils. Eosinophils are similar to neutrophils, except the cytoplasm is coarser and deeper red staining due to the presence of eosinophilic basic protein; eosinophils rarely have more than three nuclear lobes.

A significant eosinophilia is not a feature of microscopic polyarteritis.

Pulmonary eosinophilia is defined as a combination of a peripheral blood eosinophilia with an eosinophilic lung infiltrate usually manifest as shadowing on the chest X-ray.

Recognized causes of true pulmonary eosinophilia include:
- Fungi: commonly *Aspergillus fumigatus* (this consists of asthma, fleeting pulmonary infiltrates with a tendency to mucus impaction and bronchial wall damage which leads to proximal bronchiectasis.
- Drugs and toxins, e.g. tetracyclines, sulfonamides, nitrofurantoin, non-steroidal anti-inflammatory drugs, Spanish toxic oil syndrome.
- Parasites, including *Ascaris*, *Strongyloides*, *Ankylostoma*, filariae and schistosomiasis.
- Vasculitides, typically Churg–Strauss syndrome.
- Loffler's syndrome (simple pulmonary eosinophilia) – usually a self limiting illness presenting with a cough and sputum. There is a modest eosinophilia ($1–2 \times 10^9$) and fleeting peripheral pulmonary shadows.
- Eosinophilic pneumonia and prolonged pulmonary eosinophilia – a more chronic illness with extensive pulmonary disease and systemic manifestations.
- Pulmonary eosinophilia with bronchial involvement – asthma is associated with a mild eosinophilia (counts of $\sim 0.4 \times 10^9$ are not unexpected).
- Hypereosinophilic syndrome – very high eosinophil counts of $50\,000–100\,000/mm^3$: it would appear to represent a myeloproliferative state.

High eosinophil counts without pulmonary involvement can occur in:
- Eczema
- Scabies
- Pemphigus
- Pemphigoid
- Rheumatoid arthritis
- Lymphoma
- Addison's disease.

This 40-year-old woman has been referred to vascular surgeons with worsening claudication; she is a non-smoker. Her past medical history has included a myocardial infarction, hypertension and recurrent episodes of upper gastrointestinal blood loss, with no evidence of peptic ulceration at endoscopy.

What is the diagnosis?

1. Ehlers–Danlos syndrome
2. Pseudoxanthoma elasticum
3. Sickle cell disease
4. Type II hypercholesterolaemia
5. Systemic lupus erythematosus

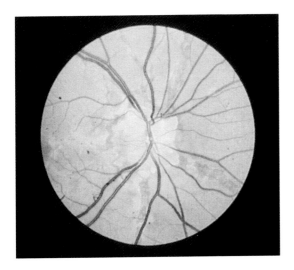

2. **Pseudoxanthoma elasticum.**

The slide shows angioid streaks. These are crack-like breaks in the collagenous and elastic portions of Bruch's membrane. (An additional and sometimes associated finding of intrapapillary drusen is also noted).*

    The history of peripheral vascular disease, coronary artery disease, hypertension and gastrointestinal haemorrhage points to a diagnosis of pseudoxanthoma elasticum. Gastrointestinal haemorrhage is a feature of Ehlers–Danlos syndrome but occlusive peripheral and coronary artery disease is not.

    Pseudoxanthoma elasticum is a hereditary disorder of elastic tissue; four distinct types are recognized: two are autosomal dominant and two autosomal recessive.

- The skin in pseudoxanthoma elasticum is typically loose, often hanging in folds, and has a chicken skin appearance with small yellow 'pseudoxanthomatous' plaques.
- Other clinical features of the disease include blue sclerae, myopia, lax joints and mitral valve prolapse.

Causes of angioid streaks
50% of patients have no underlying disorder.
    The remainder are associated with one of the following:
- Pseudoxanthoma elasticum
- Ehlers–Danlos syndrome
- Paget's disease
- Sickle cell disease.

Note: Intrapapillary drusen are traces of hyaline material seen in 0.4% of Caucasians. The lesions usually progress slowly and are associated with field defects, but macula vision is almost never affected. They are also an associated finding in eyes with angioid streaks.

This 30-year-old female patient presents with transient visual changes that last for a few seconds. She visited her optician. He informed her that she didn't need any glasses but was very concerned about the following fundal changes.

What is the diagnosis?

1. Grade IV hypertensive retinopathy
2. Proliferative diabetic retinopathy
3. Central retinal vein occlusion
4. Papilloedema
5. Optic neuritis

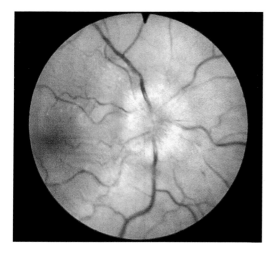

4. Papilloedema.

This shows the typical appearances of papilloedema: the disc is pink and swollen and has indistinct margins. The swollen disc is often accompanied by venous engorgement and flame-shaped haemorrhages centred around the disc.

Papilloedema is defined as swelling of the optic nerve head secondary to raised intracranial pressure.

Note: Optic disc swelling and papilloedema are terms that have been used interchangeably. It is now usual to use the term papilloedema if the optic disc swelling is secondary to raised intracranial pressure and to use the term disc swelling for all other causes of disc oedema that are not associated with raised intracranial pressure.

- An intracranial mass lesion leading to raised intracranial pressure is the diagnosis of exclusion when these appearances are detected.
- Patients will often complain of headaches, which are typically most severe in the morning and sometimes can be made worse by bending or straining. They may suddenly become nauseous and often vomit.
- In the early stages of papilloedema visual symptoms tend to be absent and visual acuity remains normal, in contrast to disc swelling due to a papillitis or optic neuritis, where there is early loss of visual acuity and a large central scotoma. Fleeting episodes of visual loss in one or both eyes can then ensue and these are virtually pathognomonic of papilloedema. Other visual changes accompanying papilloedema include gradual enlargement of the blind spot and concentric diminution of the visual fields.

The causes of papilloedema (and therefore raised intracranial pressure) include:

Space-occupying lesions	Including mass effect secondary to intracranial haemorrhage
Blockage of the ventricular system	By congenital or acquired lesions
Obstruction of CSF absorption	Damaged by meningitis, subarachnoid haemorrhage or cerebral trauma
Benign intracranial hypertension	
Diffuse cerebral oedema	Such as due to blunt head trauma
Severe hypertension	
Hypersecretion of CSF	Choroid plexus tumours (rare)

The causes of disc swelling include:

1. Raised intracranial pressure
2. Accelerated phase hypertension
3. Retinal vein thrombosis
4. Papillitis
5. Carbon dioxide retention
6. Hypoparathyroidism
7. Acute intermittent porphyria
8. Lead poisoning
9. Guillain–Barré syndrome
10. Bacterial endocarditis
11. Behçet's syndrome
12. Systemic lupus erythematosus.

This is the peripheral blood film and Perls' stain of the bone marrow from this 50-year-old man with anaemia.

What is the diagnosis?

1. Iron deficiency anaemia that has been partially treated
2. Beta thalassaemia major
3. Mixed iron or folate and B$_{12}$ deficiency
4. Sideroblastic anaemia
5. Hairy cell leukaemia

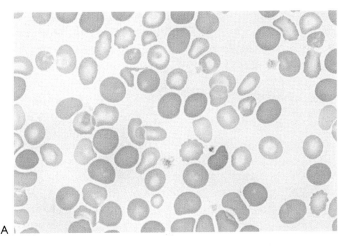

A

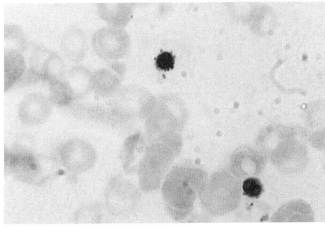

B

4. Sideroblastic anaemia.

The blood film is dimorphic and the bone marrow shows ring sideroblasts.

The differential diagnosis of a dimorphic blood film includes:
(i) sideroblastic anaemia; (ii) recent blood transfusion; (iii) treated iron deficiency; (iv) mixed iron and folate or B_{12} deficiency.

Sideroblastic anaemias are a group of disorders characterized by increased numbers of ring sideroblasts in the bone marrow. Ring sideroblasts owe their appearance to the abnormal deposits of iron in perinuclear mitochondria which form a blue-green collar around the nucleus when stained with Perls' stain. The peripheral blood film in sideroblastic anaemia is dimorphic, with a population of hypochromic microcytic cells caused by an underlying abnormality in haem synthesis. Despite the presence of this population the anaemia is commonly macrocytic.

Congenital (usually X-linked) sideroblastic anaemia is rare but may respond well to pyridoxine.

There is a wide range of causes of acquired sideroblastic anaemia. Drugs, particularly alcohol, are an important and potentially reversible cause. Most cases of acquired sideroblastic anaemia, however, are idiopathic and classified with the myelodysplastic syndromes. They usually present as a macrocytic anaemia with additional neutropenia or thrombocytopenia. If there is no response to a trial of pyridoxine, and drug-induced sideroblastic anaemia has been excluded, treatment usually consists of blood transfusion with iron chelation where appropriate

Classification of sideroblastic anaemias
- Congenital:
  — X-linked (rare).
- Acquired:
  — Idiopathic (myelodysplastic syndromes)
  — Alcohol and lead
  — Drug-induced, e.g. isoniazid, chloramphenicol
  — Rheumatoid arthritis
  — Myeloma and malignancy.

This gallium-67 scan was performed on a 24-year-old man who presented with pyrexia of unknown origin.

What is the likely diagnosis?

1. Lymphoma
2. Tuberculosis
3. Brucellosis
4. Sarcoidosis
5. Systemic lupus erythematosus

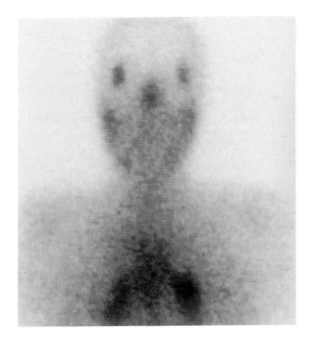

4. Sarcoidosis.

The gallium scan shows increased uptake in the salivary and lacrimal glands and hilar lymph nodes. This pattern is highly suggestive of sarcoidosis.

Sarcoidosis is a multisystem disease of unknown aetiology characterized by the presence of non-caseating granulomas. Diagnosis requires the exclusion of infections such as tuberculosis, a compatible clinical picture and if possible histology, though the latter is not always possible.

Chest X-rays may reveal hilar and paratracheal lymphadenopathy plus evidence of a mid and upper zone pulmonary infiltrate. CT scanning of the lungs may show typical hilar lymphadenopathy and thickening of the bronchovascular bundles. Lung function tests may reveal a restrictive lung defect or just a reduction in the transfer factor. Fibre-optic bronchoscopy will allow visualization of the upper airways and mucosal and transbronchial biopsies can be taken if appropriate. Bronchoalveolar lavage typically shows an increased lymphocyte count with an elevated CD4 to CD8 ratio.

All patients should have a slit-lamp examination performed to look for evidence of uveitis.

In the appropriate clinical context biopsy of the skin, muscle, synovium, parotid or meninges often yield non-caseating granulomas.

The serum ACE is raised in approximately 70% of cases. Serum immunoglobulins are often elevated in a polyclonal pattern and may be accompanied by a modest acute phase response. Liver function tests are often abnormal and reflect hepatic involvement and a liver biopsy may yield non-caseating granulomas. The serum calcium is elevated in approximately 5% and 24-hour urine calcium levels in a higher percentage.

This patient presented with a four-week history of malaise, low-grade fever and pain over the nasal bridge.

Which of the following is *not* a well-recognized complication of this disease?

1. Stridor
2. Nephrotic syndrome
3. Acute iritis
4. Aortic regurgitation
5. Non-erosive inflammatory arthritis

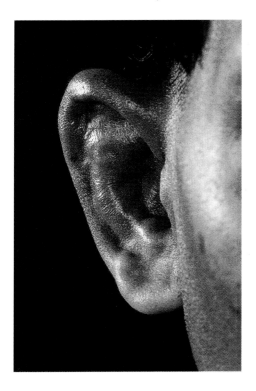

2. Nephrotic syndrome.

This is the typical appearance of inflammation of the pinna secondary to relapsing polychondritis.

Relapsing polychondritis is a multisystem disorder characterized by episodic and sometimes progressive inflammation of cartilaginous structures and tissues rich in glycosoaminoglycans. Destroyed cartilage is replaced by granulation tissue and with subsequent fibrosis there is collapse of cartilaginous structures.

Typically patients are in their forties to fifties and they have recurrent swelling and pain of the ear and/or nose (leading to collapse of the nasal bridge) associated with ocular involvement – episcleritis, conjunctivitis, scleritis and uveitis – and a non-erosive arthropathy. Episodes of inflammation are often sudden and last for days. The respiratory tract is affected in 50% of patients, leading to breakdown of the tracheal and bronchial cartilage. The larynx and upper trachea are frequently involved and subglottic narrowing is a common finding. Dysphonia, recurrent cough, stridor and shortness of breath are therefore common clinical findings.

The diagnostic criteria were set by McAdam in 1976. The presence of three or more clinical features is considered diagnostic:

- Recurrent chondritis of both auricles
- Non-erosive polyarthritis
- Chondritis of the nasal cartilage
- Inflammation of ocular structures
- Chondritis of the larynx or trachea
- Cochlear or vestibular involvement.

Aortic regurgitation is eventually seen in up to 25% of patients.

A focal glomerulonephritis has occasionally been reported but nephrotic syndrome is not a recognized complication.

Which of the following is *least* likely to be responsible for the appearance of this blood film?

1. Iron deficiency
2. Sideroblastic anaemia
3. Beta-thalassaemic trait
4. Alpha-thalassaemic trait
5. Hypothyroidism

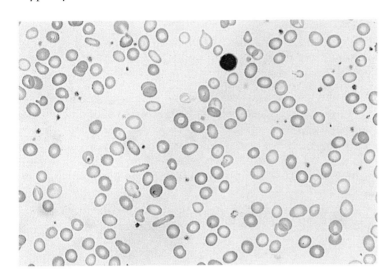

5. Hypothyroidism.

Hypothyroidism is associated with an elevated mean corpuscular volume.

The red cells are hypochromic (they are extremely pale) and microcytic (the majority are considerably smaller than the normal lymphocyte).

Hypochromic anaemias are caused by abnormal synthesis of haemoglobin and the causes are:

- Iron deficiency
- Alpha- or beta-thalassaemia
- Sideroblastic anaemia.
- Anaemia of chronic disease (the red cells are most commonly normochromic and normocytic but in 30–35% of patients they are hypochromic and microcytic).

This blood film is from a patient with iron deficiency anaemia but it is not possible to differentiate between these diagnostic possibilities without further information:

- A careful history (e.g. gastrointestinal symptoms, menorrhagia, ethnic origin, family and past medical history) and examination are essential.
- Investigation rests on assessment of iron status and haemoglobin electrophoresis if appropriate.
- Sideroblastic anaemia can only be diagnosed by a bone marrow aspirate with Perls' iron stain to look for ring sideroblasts.

This lady presented to casualty with acute pulmonary oedema.

Her pulse is 100 regular, BP 210/110 mmHg. She has dual heart sounds with no added sounds heard; auscultation of the chest reveals bilateral end-inspiratory crepitations to the midzones. She has no peripheral oedema. At fundoscopy grade III hypertensive changes are noted.

- ECG sinus, tachycardia, no acute ischaemia
- Chest X-ray consistent with pulmonary oedema.
- Hb 9 g/dL; fragmented cells seen on the blood film
- WCC 6×10^9/L
- Platelets 350×10^9/L
- Urea 18 mmol/L
- Creatinine 220 µmol/L
- Urine: protein +, no blood.

The likely diagnosis is:

1. Haemolytic uraemic syndrome
2. Rapidly progressive glomerulonephritis
3. Hypertensive heart disease
4. Renal hypertensive crisis
5. Renal artery stenosis

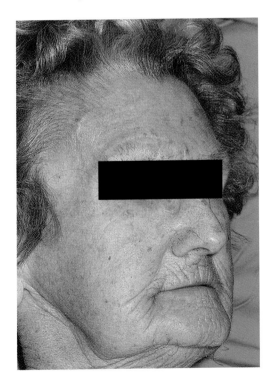

4. Renal hypertensive crisis.

The patient has classical scleroderma: She has multiple telangectasia, skin tightening and the typical beaked nose. The clinical presentation is typical of an acute scleroderma renal hypertensive crisis. This is one of the most important complications of scleroderma and is amenable to treatment, though prognosis is much better with early diagnosis and intervention. This usually occurs in people with diffuse disease within five years of diagnosis.

- It is characterized by acute onset of hypertension, >160/90 mmHg, grade III or grade IV hypertensive retinopathy, rapid deterioration in renal function and a raised plasma renin.
- A microangiopathic haemolytic anaemia is typical. Patients present with headache, pulmonary oedema, visual disturbance or seizures.
- Renal biopsy performed when the patient is stable and normotensive shows fibrinoid necrosis, mucoid or fibromucoid proliferative intimal lesions in renal arteries, particularly the arcuate and interlobular arteries. Glomerular thrombi occur eventually leading to glomerulosclerosis. The extent of glomeruli involvement is useful in predicting functional recovery.
- Patients should be managed in a high-dependency setting. Precipitous drops in blood pressure should be avoided.
- Intravenous prostacyclin and oral angiotensin-converting enzyme inhibitors are used for blood pressure control.
- Short-term haemodialysis may be necessary; some patients may require longer dialysis and peritoneal dialysis is generally well tolerated.
- While some patients remain dialysis dependent, the potential for a slow recovery of renal function over one to two years is well recognized.
- Two other important clinical points:
  - The routine use of angiotensin-converting enzyme inhibitors lessens the likelihood of scleroderma renal crisis developing.
  - High doses of prednisolone, >20 mg a day, appear to increase the risk of developing a scleroderma renal crisis and should be avoided.

Other dermatological features of systemic sclerosis include:
- Sclerodactyly
- Raynaud's phenomenon
- Calcification
- Pulp atrophy
- Ulceration
- Increased pigmentation
- Vitiligo.

This 35-year-old businessman returned six weeks ago from a holiday in Thailand. He is generally well. On examination, there is widespread lymphadenopathy and the palmar rash shown.

What is the most appropriate treatment?

1. Doxycycline
2. Symptomatic treatment only
3. i.m. procaine benzylpenicillin
4. Highly active antiretroviral therapy
5. Acyclovir

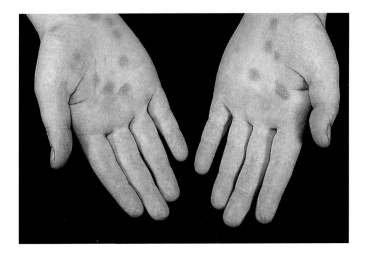

3. i.m. procaine benzylpenicillin.

The slide shows symmetrical, well-demarcated, dusky red palmar lesions typical of secondary syphilis. The lesions of secondary syphilis occur four to eight weeks after the primary lesion (chancre), which may still be present in up to a third of cases.

Clinical manifestations vary greatly. Some patients present with malaise and a widespread symmetrical macular or maculopapular, non-itchy rash (lesions crop, collarettes are present). Others present with a subtle transient eruption over the flanks. Widespread discrete non-tender lymphadenopathy is common.

Other clinical manifestations of secondary syphilis include:

1. Shallow, painless erosions of mucous membranes – snail track ulcers
2. Condylomata lata; in warm, moist areas papular lesions may coalesce to form large fleshy masses
3. Alopecia
4. Eye: uveitis, choroidoretinitis, optic neuritis
5. Locomotor: arthritis, periostitis
6. Neurological: meningitis, cranial nerve palsies
7. Rarely – hepatitis, glomerulonephritis and the nephrotic syndrome.

The diagnosis of syphilis may be confirmed by:

1. Dark-field microscopy, using material from the chancre or lymph nodes to demonstrate the spiral, motile *Treponema pallidum* organisms.
2. Serology: serological tests only become positive five to eight weeks after the original infection.

- Non-specific tests: VDRL flocculation test. Treponemal diseases including yaws, pinta and bejel will also yield positive reactions. Biological false positives are common (leprosy, connective tissue diseases) and false negatives may occur.
- Specific tests: fluorescent treponemal antibody test (FTA); *Treponema pallidum* haemagglutination assay (TPHA).

Treatment is with procaine penicillin (600mg) intramuscularly for 10 days. In cases of penicillin allergy alternatives include tetracycline or erythromycin. A mild Jarisch–Herxheimer reaction commonly complicates treatment of secondary syphilis. This reaction (fever, tachycardia, vasodilation and a flare of the existing rash) is believed to be due to release of endotoxin from the large number of organisms killed by the penicillin.

This is the peripheral blood film (slide A) and bone marrow (slide B) from a 55-year-old patient with acute renal failure.

a Which of the following describes the blood film?
1. A leukoerythroblastic blood film
2. A leukaemoid blood film
3. A dimorphic blood film
4. A microangiopathic haemolytic picture
5. Chronic myeloid leukaemia

b What is the unifying diagnosis?
1. Chronic myeloid leukaemia
2. Myeloma
3. B_{12}/folate deficiency plus iron deficiency
4. Sepsis
5. Disseminated intravascular coagulation

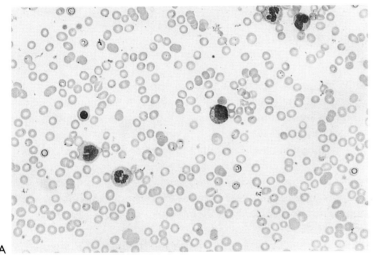

A

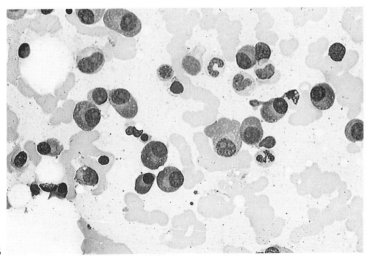

B

a 1. A leukoerythroblastic blood film
b 2. Myeloma.

The peripheral blood film shows immature nucleated red blood cells and immature myeloid cell (myelocytes): a leukoerythroblastic blood picture. Rouleaux (stacks of erythrocytes resembling a pile of coins) are also present. A leukoerythroblastic film with rouleaux formation in a patient with renal failure is highly suggestive of multiple myeloma. The diagnosis is confirmed by the plasma cell infiltrate seen in the marrow aspirate. Plasma cells are characterized by their prominent basophilic cytoplasm, eccentric nucleus and perinuclear halo. (The nucleus resembles a slice of salami.)

A leukoerythroblastic blood film is caused by disruption of normal bone marrow architecture, either by accumulation of abnormal cells (myeloma, disseminated carcinoma, Gaucher's disease) or by marrow fibrosis (myelofibrosis); it may also be seen in conditions of severe marrow stress (haemolysis, hypoxia). The underlying disorder is often only demonstrated by a bone marrow trephine, since the bone marrow aspirate is often dry when there is marrow infiltration present.

Renal impairment is present in approximately 50% of patients with myeloma at the time of presentation and often has a complex aetiology. Histologically the two commonest findings are: (i) myeloma cast nephropathy, in which dense obstructive casts cause tubular obstruction and a consequent interstitial nephritis; and (ii) a glomerular lesion caused by the deposition of amyloid and light chains. Other factors that contribute to renal impairment include hypovolaemia, hypercalcaemia, hyperuricaemia and administration of radio-iodine contrast media.

Criteria for diagnosing myeloma major: (a) plasmacytoma on biopsy; (b) >30% of plasma cells on bone marrow biopsy; (c) monoclonal band on electrophoresis >35 g/L for IgG, 20 g/L IgA, or >1.0 g of light chains excreted in the urine per day.

Criteria for diagnosing myeloma minor: (a) 10–30% of plasma cells on bone marrow biopsy; (b) abnormal monoclonal band but less than above; (c) lytic bone lesions; and (d) immune paresis.

What is the most likely underlying diagnosis?

1. Rheumatoid arthritis
2. Ankylosing spondylitis
3. Reiter's syndrome
4. Systemic lupus erythematosus
5. Crohn's disease

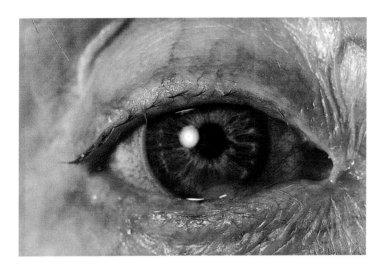

1. Rheumatoid arthritis.

The typical appearance of peripheral corneal thinning is easily seen. This is characterized by gradual resorption of peripheral corneal tissue, leaving the central part intact. This condition is sometimes called corneal melt or contact lens cornea, as the appearance can resemble a contact lens placed on the eye when it affects a larger part of the corneal circumference.

Rheumatoid arthritis is the commonest disorder to affect the peripheral cornea. It can be the first manifestation of systemic disease but is more often associated with other ocular complications associated with rheumatoid arthritis such as a sicca syndrome, scleritis and episcleritis. Systemic therapy with corticosteroids and cytotoxics is often required. Surgery in the form of keratoplasty is often needed.

The other multisystem disorders that can affect the cornea are:
- Systemic lupus erythematosus
- Wegener's granulomatosis
- Polyarteritis nodosa
- Relapsing polychondritis.

Question 68

This 25-year-old man presents with a three-month history of arthralgia, myalgia, malaise, sore throat and a fever. His condition has not improved with three separate courses of antibiotics.

Clinical examination was unremarkable other than for the rash shown.

Investigations:

Hb	11.9 g/dL
MCV	87 fL
WCC	15×10^9 (90% neutrophils)
Platelets	600×10^9/L
ESR	95 mm in the first hour
CRP	76 mg/L
Urea and electrolyte	Normal
LDH	
LFTs	Mild transaminitis

Which of the following tests is most likely to help confirm your clinical diagnosis?

1. ANA
2. ANCA
3. Blood film
4. Ferritin
5. Liver ultrasound

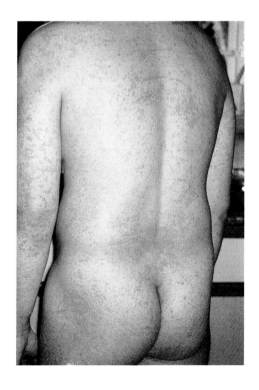

4. Ferritin.

The clinical diagnosis is adult Still's disease, an important part of the differential diagnosis of a pyrexia of unknown origin (PUO).

- The classical triad of Still's disease is fever (temperature spikes of >39°C), an oligoarthritis and an evanescent (present during the raised temperature) salmon-coloured rash.
- The fever is often only present in the early morning or late afternoon, between which the patient is apyrexial and often feels well.
- The rash of Still's disease may be subtle, is maculopapular and distributed over the trunk, arms and legs.
- Joints involved include knees, wrists, ankles, proximal interphalangeal joints and the metacarpophalangeal joints.
- Other clinical features include lymphadenopathy, splenomegaly, hepatomegaly and pericarditis.
- The ESR and CRP are elevated. Still's disease is characterized by a markedly elevated ferritin; often values in the thousands are recorded. (The reason for this elevation is not known.)
- A normochromic anaemia, and an associated neutrophil leukocytosis, are common.
- A mild transaminitis is present in 80% of patients.
- Treatment consists of non-steroidal anti-inflammatories, although corticosteroids are often required.

Other points when considering the causes of a PUO:
- Consider infection, neoplasia (lymphomas) and connective tissue diseases.
- A PUO is due to infection in one-third to one-half of cases, underlying malignancy in another third and autoimmune disease in a quarter.
- Drug fevers should also always be considered.

The feature shown in the slide is noted in a 67-year-old man. He is most likely:

1. Symptomatic from a retro-orbital headache
2. Complaining of transient visual obscurations
3. Asymptomatic
4. To have permanent vision loss in the eye
5. Having attacks of amaurosis fugax

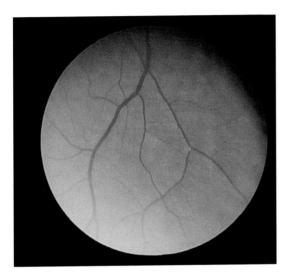

3. Asymptomatic.

Hollenhorst plaques, which are cholesterol emboli, are seen here. These are intermittent showers of minute, bright, refractile, golden to yellow crystals, often located at arteriolar bifurcations. They rarely cause significant obstruction to the retinal arterioles and are frequently asymptomatic since the blood tends to flow around the emboli.

Cholesterol emboli are associated with underlying severe atherosclerotic disease, particularly of the carotids.

Angiography, carotid operation, anticoagulation or trauma may precede the embolization of cholesterol crystals.

A serious complication of generalized cholesterol embolization is renal involvement, leading to renal failure. Patients may have livedo reticularis as a result of cholesterol emboli lodging in skin vessels.

What is the likely diagnosis?

1. Testicular feminization syndrome
2. Klinefelter's syndrome
3. Constitutional delayed puberty
4. Congenital adrenal hyperplasia
5. Marfan's syndrome

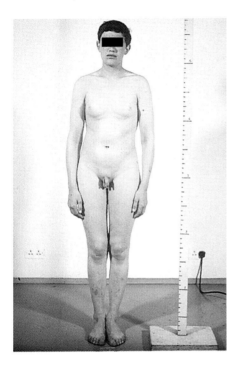

2. Klinefelter's syndrome.

This is the classical appearance of **Klinefelter's syndrome**: tall stature with gynaecomastia and small external genitalia. Patients are infertile and spermatozoa are never present; they can, however, have erections and ejaculate. Other features include mental retardation and an increased incidence of both breast and testicular cancers. Chromosomal analysis will reveal the classical XXY chromosomal complement.

Buccal smear cells from the buccal mucosa will be chromatin positive; i.e. there is a small darkly staining body (the Barr body) inside the nuclear membrane which is present in normal females but not normal (XY) males. Its presence indicates there are two X chromosomes in the nucleus. The Lyon hypothesis states: 'twelve days after fertilization one X chromosome in every cell of a female fetus becomes inactive; which one of the X chromosomes becomes inactive is decided at random'. The Barr body represents the condensed inactive X chromosome.

The mainstay of treatment for the hypogonadal male is androgen replacement. Bone density should be regularly monitored.

Other notes:
Testicular feminization syndrome: patients are phenotypically female. The condition is due to either complete or incomplete androgen insensitivity. In the complete form patients usually present after puberty with normal breast development, scanty axillary and pubic hair and a blind ending vagina. In the incomplete form there is more virilization, which is manifest as clitoral enlargement and labial fusion.

Constitutional delayed puberty: these are normal adolescents who have relatively short stature, delayed puberty and bone age, and a height prognosis appropriate in relation to their parents. It presents far more commonly in boys than girls and is the commonest cause of delayed puberty in boys, Turner's syndrome being the commonest in girls.

This blood film was taken from a 26-year-old African male who presented with lethargy, fever and cervical lymphadenopathy.
    What treatment would you recommend?

1. Sodium stibogluconate
2. Praziquantel
3. Suramin
4. Tiabendazole
5. Diethylcarbamazine

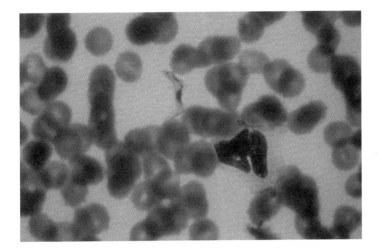

3. Suramin.

The slide shows an undulated trypanosome with its characteristic undulated membrane, anterior flagellum, prominent nucleus and darkly staining kinetoplast.

African trypanosomiasis occurs in two forms:

1. West African or Gambian sleeping sickness is caused by infection with *Trypanosoma brucei gambiense*.
2. East African or Rhodesian sleeping sickness is caused by infection with *Trypanosoma brucei rhodesiense*.

West African sleeping sickness is primarily a human infection, while the East African form is a zoonosis. Both types are spread by the tsetse fly.

Gambian sleeping sickness: two to six weeks after a tsetse fly bite a localized chancroid develops. Several weeks later systemic trypanosomiasis develops. The patient has fever, malaise, cervical lymphadenopathy and splenomegaly. After a variable period of time the fever subsides, the lymphadenopathy regresses and the patient becomes asymptomatic. During this asymptomatic period invasion of the central nervous system occurs. Clinical features include a change in personality, daytime sleepiness, headache, backache, extrapyramidal signs and severe itching. Cardiac involvement is rare and mild. Finally the patient becomes stuporose and dies of secondary bacterial infections.

Rhodesian sleeping sickness is similar but the clinical course is more rapid; cardiac involvement is often severe and responsible for death. Haemolytic anaemia, thrombocytopenia and disseminated intravascular coagulation are commoner in the Rhodesian form.

Serum IgM levels are raised in both types. CNS involvement is associated with a lymphocytic CNS and trypanosomes may be found in the CSF in 50% of cases.

The diagnosis is confirmed by finding trypanosomes in the blood of early cases of Rhodesian sleeping sickness. Trypanosomes are less commonly found in the Gambian form, so the diagnosis is made by gland puncture and aspiration.

Drug	Indication
Suramin	Early-stage disease but poor CNS penetration (melarsoprol is used for late stages with CNS involvement.)
Sodium stibogluconate	Visceral leishmaniasis
Tiabendazole	*Strongyloides* and cutaneous and visceral larva migrans
Praziquantel	Schistosomiasis
Diethylcarbamazine	Filarial infections

This 25-year-old woman is being treated for acute leukaemia. She has complained of blurred vision.

What is the most likely diagnosis?

1. Toxoplasmosis choroidoretinitis
2. *Toxocara* choroidoretinitis
3. *Candida* ophthalmitis
4. Cytomegalovirus choroidoretinitis
5. Choroidal tubercules

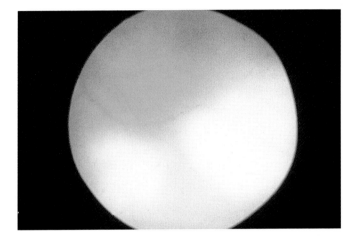

3. *Candida* ophthalmitis.

The slide shows white fluffy intravitreal ball-like lesions characteristic of *Candida* endophthalmitis. Fundal candida may also manifest as yellow-white chorioretinal lesions or in chronic infections as white vitreoretinal scars, often associated with traction. (Differential diagnosis: reactivation of toxoplasmosis.)

Disseminated candidiasis (*Candida albicans* and *Candida tropicalis*) occurs in patients who are immunosuppressed, debilitated or receiving parenteral nutrition, and in intravenous heroin abusers.

The diagnosis is usually made clinically. Blood cultures are positive in only 50% of cases; however, it is often possible to isolate *Candida* from cutaneous lesions or bone marrow aspirates. Serological tests are of limited value in clinical management.

Treatment options include oral flucytosine with oral ketoconazole or i.v. amphotericin.

This small bowel biopsy was performed on a 24-year-old man who presented with weight loss and diarrhoea.

What treatment would you prescribe?

1. Profloxacin
2. Vancomycin
3. Spiramycin
4. Metronidazole
5. Tiabendazole

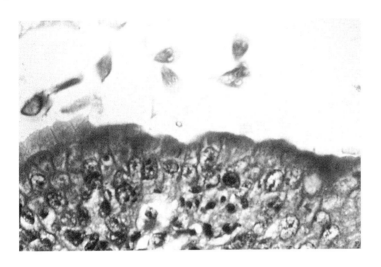

4. Metronidazole.

The slide shows *Giardia lamblia* with associated small bowel villous atrophy.

Giardia lamblia is an anaerobic flagellate parasite with two nuclei that infects the small bowel.

- It has a worldwide distribution (common in the tropics and endemic in Eastern Europe). The most important modes of transmission are food contamination with cysts or inadequately treated water.
- Man-to-man spread is also recognized in homosexuals.
- The incubation period is approximately two weeks.
- Giardiasis presents with anorexia, weight loss and acute or chronic diarrhoea with watery, yellow foul-smelling stools.
- The diagnosis is usually confirmed by finding faecal cysts. Alternatively the trophozoites may be isolated from small bowel aspirates or be visibly attached to the surface of epithelial cells in a small bowel biopsy.
- The amount of villous atrophy varies considerably; however, a completely atrophic biopsy should raise the possibility of underlying coeliac disease.
- A small percentage of gluten-sensitive patients present when mild diarrhoea is made worse by the additional insult of an intestinal infection.
- Malabsorption of fat, B_{12} and D-xylose is present in severe cases. Lactulose intolerance may occur and persist for some time after treatment.
- Treatment is with metronidazole and symptoms should settle within 3–10 days.

Question 74

Which of the following investigations would be most useful in reaching a diagnosis?

1. Thyroid autoantibodies
2. Insulin stress test
3. Serum IGF-1
4. Glucose tolerance test
5. Blood cultures

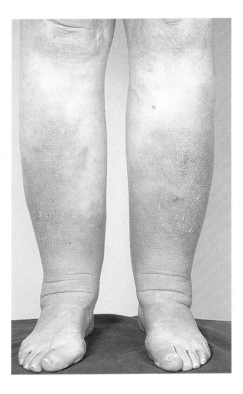

1. Thyroid autoantibodies.

The slide shows the typical appearances of pre-tibial myxoedema. The skin is symmetrically thickened and reddish-brown, with a *peau d'orange* appearance. Variants include plaque forms, nodular forms and an elephantiasic form.

Pre-tibial myxoedema is most commonly associated with ophthalmic Graves' disease, although it can also be seen with thyroid acropachy.

- As with ophthalmic Graves' disease, pre-tibial myxoedema may be found in the absence of other features of autoimmune thyroid disease, and can appear after treatment of hyperthyroidism in Graves' disease.
- Biopsy of areas of pre-tibial myxoedema is not recommended as lesions heal slowly, often with keloid formation. Histology of affected skin shows infiltration of the subcutaneous tissue with glycosaminoglycans.
- Deposits tend to persist despite biochemical control of hyperthyroidism; treatment with topical steroids may be effective.

What is the diagnosis?

1. Lichen planus
2. Dermatitis herpetiformis
3. Pustular psoriasis
4. Scabies
5. Porphyria cutanea tarda

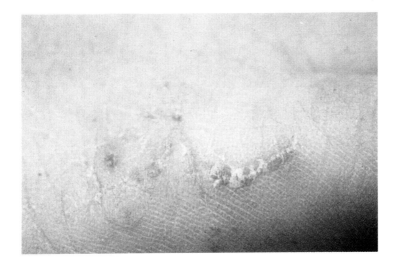

4. Scabies.

The slide shows a typical burrow caused by the mite *Sarcoptes scabei*.

- Female mites, which can survive 36 hours away from the host, burrow into the epidermis and lay their eggs. Burrows are often sparse but may be seen in the web spaces of the fingers and the flexor aspects of the wrists. Burrows do not occur above the neckline, except in infants and immunosuppressed patients. Pruritus, worse at night, develops four to six weeks after infection, when the patient develops a hypersensitivity reaction to the mite or its fomites, leading to widespread excoriations. Urticarial papules generally only occur around the penis, buttocks, areolae and umbilicus.
- The diagnosis is confirmed by identifying an adult female, obtained from an intradermal burrow with a needle. If burrows are difficult to find Cullen and Childers' test may be employed: topical tetracycline is taken up into burrows and will fluoresce yellow under Wood's light.
- Treatment should be given to the index case and all close contacts. Agents used include lindane, malathion and permethrin. Older agents, such as benzyl benzoate, should be avoided in children.
- Secondary bacterial infection, typically *Staphylococcus* or *Streptococcus*, is common, especially in the tropics; appropriate antibiotics should be given.
- A highly contagious variant, Norwegian scabies, occurs in institutions and immunosuppressed patients and may lead to a hypertrophic psoriaform rash. Ivermectin has been used with good effect.

This patient presented to her GP complaining of persistent headaches. How would you confirm the diagnosis?

1. Skull X-ray
2. Prolactin levels
3. Insulin stress test
4. Oral glucose tolerance test with measurement of growth hormone levels
5. Cranial magnetic resonance imaging

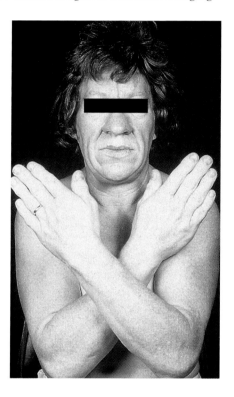

4. Oral glucose tolerance test with measurement of growth hormone levels.

Growth hormone (GH) levels would be elevated and fail to suppress (<4 mU/L) during the test. The patient has acromegaly due to excess GH secretion.

- Serum insulin-like growth factor 1 (IGF-1) is an effective and reliable screen for acromegaly and would be the first test to request if the diagnosis was suspected.
- The prolactin levels are also often elevated.
- A lateral skull X-ray will show enlargement of the pituitary fossa in 90% of cases. Computed tomography and better still magnetic resonance imaging can identify a microadenoma and show the extent of tumour growth.

Clinical features of acromegaly include:
— Thickened greasy skin
— Enlargement of the skeleton with alteration in ring, hat and shoe size, etc.
— Prognathism
— Hyperhydrosis
— Hirsutism
— Diabetes mellitus
— Hypertension
— Cardiomyopathy
— Visceromegaly
— Entrapment neuropathy (e.g. carpal tunnel syndrome)
— Arthropathy, mainly of the hips and knees
— Proximal myopathy
— Hypercalcuria.

- *Local effects of tumour include*: pressure on optic chiasm, resulting in an upper quadrant bitemporal hemianopia – all patients should have visual fields plotted; lateral extension into cavernous sinus causing IIIrd, IVth or Vth cranial nerve palsies; headaches are common and are caused by local stretching of the dura.
- *Systemically*, patients often suffer from sleep apnoea; features related to high prolactin levels or hypopituitarism may be present. Cardiovascular complications are a major source of morbidity. There is an increased risk of colorectal cancer.
- *Treatment*: Overall life expectancy is improved if the mean serum GH is less then 5 mu/L and there is normal IGF-1.
- *Treatment options include*: bromocriptine – a dopamine agonist; somatostatin analogues, e.g. octreotide; transsphenoidal hypophysectomy or transfrontal craniotomy followed by external radiation; external radiotherapy alone; yttrium-90 implants.

This young male was admitted with fever and tachypnoea.
The most appropriate treatment would be:

1. i.v. benzylpenicillin and clarythromycin
2. Oral ciprofloxacin
3. Co-trimoxazole
4. Triple therapy for tuberculosis
5. i.v. amphotericin

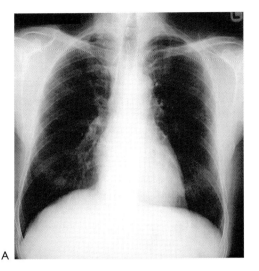

A

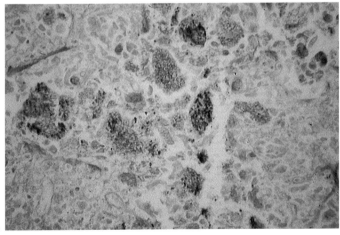

B

3. Co-trimoxazole.

The chest X-ray is normal but the lung biopsy shows the presence of *Pneumocystis carinii* cysts.

Pneumocystis pneumonia occurs almost exclusively in immunocompromised patients.

- It typically presents with a gradual history of increasing shortness of breath, a non-productive cough, tachypnoea and low-grade fever.
- At this early stage there are often no clinical signs and the chest X-ray is normal. Marked hypoxia is common and precedes radiological changes by several days. In advanced cases the chest X-ray shows diffuse bilateral alveolar shadowing.
- The diagnosis is confirmed by finding the organisms in alveolar washings or, more dependably, in a lung biopsy. *Pneumocystis* stains poorly with conventional stains; therefore silver stains are essential to show the organisms clustered in the alveoli and being phagocytosed by macrophages.
- Antibodies are not useful in making the diagnosis since most normal people have antibodies by 4 years of age, following subclinical infection.
- Co-trimoxazole is the drug of choice; pentamidine isothionate or clindamycin and primaquine are alternatives. Untreated cases of *Pneumocystis* pneumonia have a fatality rate of approximately 100%; effective treatment reduces the fatality rate to 25%.

Which form of hyperlipidaemia is this abnormality most commonly associated with?

1. Type IIa
2. Type III
3. Type IIb
4. Type I
5. Type IV

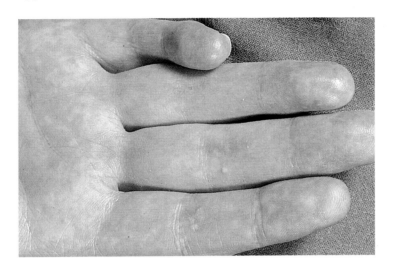

2. Type III.

The slide shows the typical appearance of palmar xanthomata. These are characteristic of **type III hyperlipoproteinaemia (broad-beta disease)**. This occurs in 1:5000 individuals and is characterized by high circulating levels of IDL (intermediate-density lipoproteins) leading to high serum cholesterol and triglyceride levels. It is generally thought to be an autosomal recessive condition due to a mutation or polymorphism affecting the apoE gene. It is rare in pre-menopausal women because oestrogens enhance hepatic uptake of IDL. Striate palmar xanthomata are present in 50% of individuals and typically take the form of orange-yellow seed-like lesions within the palmar and finger creases. Tuboeruptive xanthomata may also be present; these are yellow nodular lesions over the tuberosities. Accelerated atherosclerosis of the femoral and tibial arteries leading to vascular claudication and premature coronary disease is also often present.

(Please refer to the table in the answer to question 22.)

The chemotherapeutic agent of choice is:

1. Diethylcarbamazine
2. i.v. amphotericin
3. Tiabendazole
4. Praziquantel
5. Sodium stibogluconate

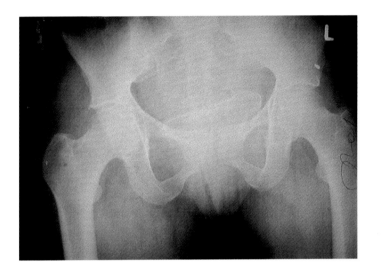

4. Praziquantel.

There is calcification within the bladder wall caused by chronic infection with *Schistosoma haematobium*.

Schistosomiasis is caused by trematodes. There are three common species:

1. *S. haematobium* (Africa and the Middle East)
2. *S. mansoni* (Africa, South America and the Caribbean)
3. *S. japonicum* (Orient and South East Asia).

- The fresh-water larvae (cercariae) penetrate the skin and migrate to the lungs and then the liver, where they mature. The adult worms migrate to their final habitat: in the case of *S. mansoni* and *S. japonicum* the venules of the intestines and in the case of *S. haematobium* the venules of the ureter and bladder. Eggs produced reach fresh water via the urine or faeces and hatch into ciliated miracidia, which infect particular species of snails (intermediate hosts) to complete the cycle.
- Penetration of the skin by cercariae may cause a hypersensitivity rash (swimmer's itch). Three to eight weeks after infection, acute schistosomiasis develops with headache, fever, myalgia, hepatosplenomegaly, lymphadenopathy, urticaria and eosinophilia. Symptoms of acute schistosomiasis are common with *S. japonicum*, rare with *S. mansoni* and extremely rare with *S. haematobium*.

There are a number of complications associated with chronic schistosomiasis and this depends on the species:

1. Urinary (*S. haematobium*): ureteric and bladder fibrosis; bladder wall calcification; carcinoma of the bladder; hydronephrosis; renal failure; haemospermia in men and sterility in women.
2. Liver (*S. mansoni*, *S. japonicum*): intrahepatic portal hypertension; hepatosplenomegaly; and the development of portal-systemic collaterals. Liver function tests are usually normal. It is debatable whether schistosomiasis alone causes cirrhosis or liver failure.
3. Lung (severe disease is a feature of *S. mansoni* and *S. japonicum*): pulmonary hypertension and cor pulmonale.
4. Central nervous system: *S. japonicum* typically affects the brain and is a common cause of focal epilepsy; it is rarely responsible for a generalized encephalitic illness. *S. mansoni* and *S. japonicum* may affect the spinal cord, causing a transverse myelitis.
5. Systemic amyloidosis.

- The definitive diagnosis is made by finding viable eggs in the urine or faeces, or by biopsying the bladder wall or rectum.
- The eggs of each species are distinctive: *S. mansoni*: ellipsoidal eggs with a lateral spine; *S. haematobium*: ellipsoidal eggs with a terminal spine; and *S. japonicum*: spheroidal eggs with a small knob.
- Praziquantel is the drug of choice; following treatment many chronic and apparently irreversible lesions will improve.

The lesions on this man's foot have developed slowly and are now painful and itchy.
What is the diagnosis?

1. Lichen planus
2. Kaposi's sarcoma
3. Stasis dermatitis
4. Lymphoma
5. Secondary syphilis

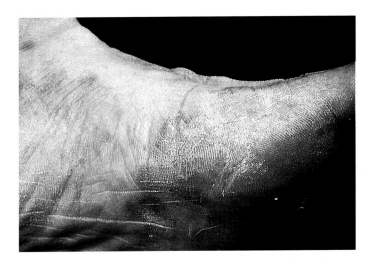

2. **Kaposi's sarcoma.**

Kaposi's sarcoma is the commonest malignancy seen in HIV disease. It most commonly occurs in a widespread symmetrical distribution over the trunk, face, extremities and oral cavity.

- It typically consists of rapidly progressive macules, patches, nodules, plaques and tumours.
- Lesions typically progress to become oval or elongated in shape and follow the lines of skin cleavage. They vary in colour from pink to red, purple or brown and can at different stages be confused with purpura, haemangiomas, naevi, pityriasis rosea, secondary syphilis, lichen planus, basal cell carcinoma and melanoma.
- AIDS-related Kaposi's can disseminate to local lymph nodes, the gastrointestinal tract, the central nervous system, lung, liver, spleen and testes.
- Chemotherapy with vinblastine is useful for early disease; late or aggressive disease can be treated with combination regimens including alpha-interferon. Radiotherapy may be used for skin and pulmonary lesions and lymphadenopathy that is causing pressure symptoms.

This is the peripheral blood from a 25-year-old diplomat with fever. Which of the following treatment options would you choose?

1. Intravenous ciprofloxacin
2. Intravenous quinine
3. Oral tetracycline
4. Diethylcarbamazine
5. Exchange transfusion

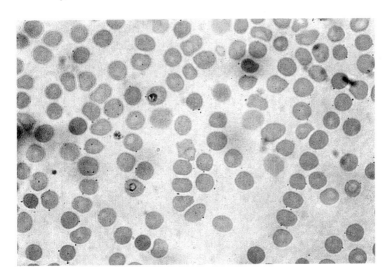

2. Intravenous quinine.

There are numerous ring forms and the diagnosis is **Plasmodium falciparum** malaria. Parasitaemia greater than 0.5% usually indicates falciparum malaria. Note the absence of platelets on the blood film.

Thrombocytopenia is very common in both falciparum and vivax malaria. Malaria must be excluded in any patient with fever who has returned from a malarious zone. There is increasing chloroquine resistance worldwide and a detailed travel history is critical. If the patient comes from an area where chloroquine resistance has been documented or is suspected, treatment with quinine should be commenced as soon as possible. Quinine therapy may produce cinchonism: tinnitus, giddiness, tremulousness and blurred vision. Hypogylcaemia may be a feature of severe falciparum malaria and can complicate quinine treatment. Quinine can rarely cause arrhythmias and thrombocytopenia.

This patient has normal T_4, T_3 and TSH.
   What is the diagnosis?

1. Orbital cellulitis
2. Wegener's granulomatosis
3. Cavernous sinus thrombosis
4. Carotico-cavernous fistula
5. Ophthalmic Graves' disease

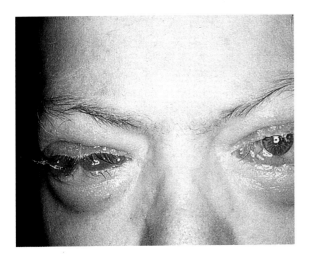

5. Ophthalmic Graves' disease.

The clinical features shown on this slide are:
- Proptosis
- Bilateral chemosis and oedema of the lids.

Sometimes this is called malignant Graves' disease – this refers to the serious risk of visual loss.

Lid lag, retraction and external ophthalmoplegia are the other common signs of thyroid eye disease. Complications include corneal ulceration, keratitis, optic nerve compression and ophthalmoplegia with diplopia. Compression of the optic nerve is often associated with only mild proptosis and may present with loss of visual acuity, field defects, colour loss or disc swelling.

Ophthalmic Graves' disease may occur in hypothyroid, euthyroid or hyperthyroid patients. Overall, 70% of patients have some evidence of thyroid gland dysfunction. The condition is usually bilateral but may be asymmetrical or unilateral. Histology shows infiltration of the external ocular muscles with lymphocytes and oedema. Circulating antibodies to ocular muscle, found in many patients, have a disputed role in pathogenesis.

The swollen muscles may be visualized by CT/MRI scanning, allowing a firm diagnosis to be made.

The differential diagnosis of asymmetrical or unilateral proptosis includes:

1. Ophthalmic Graves' disease
2. Neoplasia
3. Cavernous sinus thrombosis
4. Carotico-cavernous fistula
5. Orbital cellulitis
6. Wegener's granulomatosis.

Note: Proptosis that is asymmetrical by more than 5 mm may suggest a cause other than Graves' ophthalmopathy.

This 65-year-old Indian man presented with fever, night sweats and weight loss.

The most likely diagnosis is:

1. Tuberculous abscess
2. Secondary carcinoma of the rib
3. Calabar swelling of *Loa loa*
4. Hydatid disease
5. Leishmaniasis

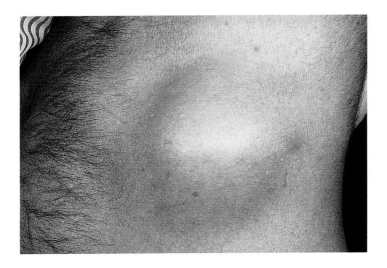

1. Tuberculous abscess.

This is a large tuberculous cold abscess. The diagnosis may be confirmed by aspiration of pus with Ziehl–Neelsen staining and culture.

Tuberculosis is treated with an initial phase using at least three drugs and a continuation phase using two drugs in fully sensitive cases.

Initial phase
This should be continued for two months. This is designed to reduce the bacterial load quickly and prevent the emergence of drug-resistant strains.

Treatment of choice is isoniazid, rifampicin, pyrazinamide and ethambutol. Ethambutol can be omitted from the regimen if the patient is not immunocompromised, has not previously been treated, and has not been in contact with possible multi-drug-resistant strains of TB. (If susceptibility results are not available full treatment should be continued.)

Continuation phase
Treatment should be continued for another four months with rifampicin and isoniazid.

Other notes:
- Streptomycin is rarely used in the UK; it can be used if resistance to isoniazid is established before treatment starts
- The standard regimen may be used in pregnancy.
- Isoniazid, rifampicin and pyrazinamide are associated with liver toxicity. Hepatic function should be checked before drugs are started.
- Renal function should also be checked: Streptomycin and ethambutol should be avoided in patients with renal impairment.
- Visual acuity should be checked before the commencement of ethambutol.
- All cases of TB require notification.

This 40-year-old Nigerian man presented with bilateral foot drop. He had palpable common peroneal and supraorbital nerves.

What is the diagnosis?

1. Lepromatous leprosy
2. Secondary syphilis
3. Secondary amyloidosis
4. Tuberculoid leprosy
5. Diffuse cutaneous *Leishmania*

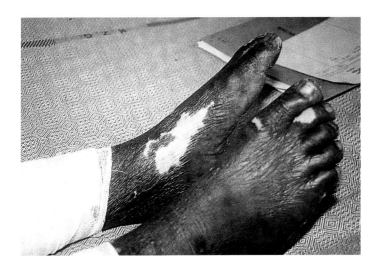

4. Tuberculoid leprosy.

The combination of hypopigmented lesions and thickened peripheral nerves is typical of the tuberculoid spectrum of leprosy.

Leprosy is caused by the acid-fast intracellular bacillus *Mycobacterium leprae*. The pattern of clinical disease is determined by the host's immune response. In tuberculoid lesions there is a strong cell-mediated response and *M. leprae* are rarely seen; in contrast, the cell-mediated response is poor in lepromatous leprosy and bacilli are abundant. The lepromin skin test, a measure of cell-mediated immunity, is strongly positive in tuberculoid but is negative in lepromatous leprosy.

- Patients with tuberculoid leprosy usually have one to three cutaneous lesions. Typically these are large and annular, with a raised outer edge and a hypopigmented centre. Alternatively, as in this case, hypopigmented macules may occur. The tuberculoid skin lesions are classically anaesthetic, anhidrotic and have lost hair. Peripheral nerve enlargement is common, particularly in the borderline tuberculoid group.
- Diagnosis is confirmed histologically. Tuberculoid lesions contain granulomas but almost no bacilli. Caseation is not a feature of tuberculoid skin granulomas but may be present in nerve lesions. The lepromin skin test is positive.
- Patients should receive at least two chemotherapeutic agents, since resistance to dapsone is increasing. Currently the recommended treatment of tuberculoid (pauci-bacterial) leprosy is daily dapsone and monthly rifampicin for six months. Clofazimine, protionamide and ethionamide have also been used.

Note:
- Triple therapy with dapsone, rifampicin and clofazimine is recommended for lepromatous leprosy.
- Leprosy is the commonest cause of peripheral nerve thickening. It can also develop in direct peripheral nerve injury, amyloidosis, neurofibromatosis and hereditary motor and sensory neuropathy.

This 25-year-old soldier presented with fever, arthralgia, and a diastolic murmur.

What is the dermatological diagnosis?

1. Erythema multiforme
2. Erythema marginatum
3. Erythema nodosum
4. Erythema chronicum migrans
5. Erythema ab igne

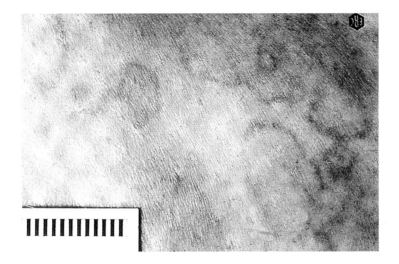

2. Erythema marginatum.

The rash is typical of erythema marginatum. This gives the patient two major criteria for the diagnosis of rheumatic fever.

These are the revised Duckett Jones criteria. There should be evidence of a recent streptococcal infection plus two major or one major and two minor criteria:

- Evidence of a recent streptococcal infection:
  - History of scarlet fever
  - Positive throat swab
  - Increase in ASOT >200 u/ml
  - Increase in DNase B titre.
- Major criteria
  - *Carditis*: tachycardia, new murmur, pericardial friction rub, CCF, cardiomegaly
  - *Subcutaneous nodules*: small, mobile, painless nodules on the extensor surfaces of the joints and spine.
  - *Erythema marginatum*: a geographical-type rash with red raised edges and a clear centre occurring mainly on the trunk, thighs and arms
  - *Arthritis*: a migratory flitting polyarthritis usually affecting the larger joints
  - *Sydenham's chorea*: unilateral or bilateral involuntary semi-purposeful movements. May be preceded by a psychiatric change.
- Minor criteria
  - Fever
  - Raised ESR or CRP
  - Arthralgia (but not if arthritis is a major criterion)
  - Prolonged P–R interval (but not if carditis is a major criterion)
  - Previous rheumatic fever.

Treatment: All patients should be given penicillin (or an alternative if penicillin allergic) during an acute attack to eradicate the streptococcal infection. High-dose aspirin is used during acute infection; steroids may be used for severe cases.

The most important point is prevention of subsequent infection with rheumatogenic strains of streptococci. Traditionally, this disease is found in children between the ages of 5 and 15, and a monthly injection of 1.2 million units of benzathine penicillin G provides effective prophylaxis. Prophylaxis is given until the age of 20, or for at least five years.

What is the clinical diagnosis?

1. Onchocerciasis
2. *Loa loa*
3. *Wuchereria bancrofti*
4. Larva currens
5. *Dracunculosis*

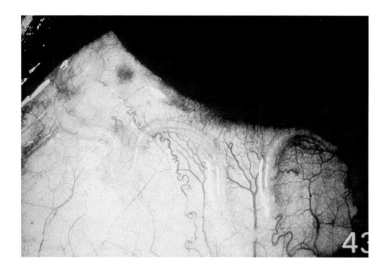

2. *Loa loa*.

This is the *Loa loa* worm migrating through the conjunctiva.

Loa loa is a filarial parasite of humans occurring in parts of west and central Africa. Infection is transmitted by infected bloodsucking flies (red fly or *chrysops*); the worms live and move in the connective tissues. Gradually the worms penetrate the deeper fascial planes and about five months after the initial bite microfilariae enter the bloodstream. One year after infection the worms have entered the deep viscera and lungs. Transient painful swellings of the limbs can occur (Calabar swellings) as the worms migrate. They can also be seen journeying through the skin, particularly of the fingers, scalp, penis, eyelids and conjunctivae. Angioedema and eosinophilia are common associated findings. Treatment is with diethylcarbamazine.

Other notes:
Dracunculosis occurs due to chronic infection with a large nematode, the guinea worm (*Dracunculus medinensis*).

Larva currens refers to the migration of *Strongyloides* under the skin. Strongyloidiasis is a nematode infection that causes diarrhoea and malabsorption. The initial symptoms are a very itchy rash at the site of infection, which is usually the foot. The larvae can then be seen migrating through the skin.

Onchocerciasis is a filarial infection of the eye transmitted by a buffalo gnat. The microfilaria are generally not present in the blood but reside in connective tissues, lymphatics and around the eye. The most significant complication is the keratitis, iritis and choroiditis that can occur early in the infection, leading to the alternative name 'river blindness'. Ivermectin is the treatment of choice.

Wuchereria bancrofti is a filarial infection that invades the lymphatics and can cause elephantiasis.

What is the diagnosis?

1. Myelinated nerve fibres
2. Drusen
3. *Candida* ophthalmitis
4. Toxoplasmosis
5. *Toxocara*

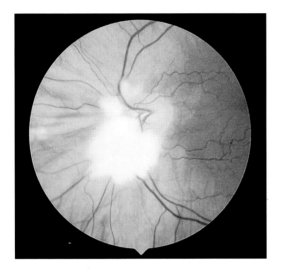

1. Myelinated nerve fibres.

There are bright white, irregular, flared, feather-like patches extending from the optic disc. This is the typical appearance of myelinated (or medullated) nerve fibres that appear brilliantly white in contrast to the red background of the fundus. Normally nerve fibres do not have myelin sheaths beyond the lamina cribrosa but in these cases they are present. The defect is present from birth and is accompanied by a corresponding field defect.

Other notes: drusen appear as multiple, discrete, round, yellow-white dots of variable size scattered around the macula. These are abnormal accumulations in the retinal pigment epithelium basement membrane (Bruch's membrane). Around the optic disc they appear as bright areas that may be calcified and they can be confused with papilloedema.

This 32-year-old male presented with a one-week history of cough, shortness of breath and feverish symptoms. He is known to be HIV positive and has been stable on antiretroviral medication. He is treated at another hospital and was routinely reviewed three weeks previously and told all was well.

His chest X-ray was taken in the accident and emergency department. What is the most likely diagnosis?

1. *Pneumocystis carinii* pneumonia
2. Pneumococcal pneumonia
3. *Legionella* pneumonia
4. Atypical mycobacterial pneumonia
5. Tuberculosis

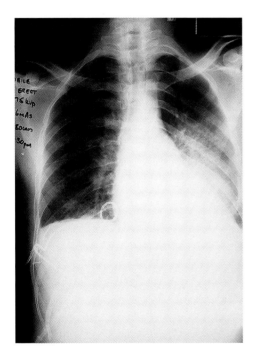

2. Pneumococcal pneumonia.

The most likely organism is streptococcal infection. This is the organism that is most commonly responsible for community-acquired pneumonia and it characteristically leads to lobar consolidation: this chest X-ray shows left lower lobe consolidation. (There is loss of clarity of the left hemidiaphragm.)

Although he has HIV there is no suggestion that he is currently immunocompromised; the usual and more common bacterial causes are still more frequently encountered in these patients than 'atypical pathogens'.

Differential diagnosis of chest infiltrates in immunocompromised patients:

Infiltrate	Infectious	Non-infectious
Localized	Common bacterial pathogens, legionella, mycobacteria	Local haemorrhage or embolism
Nodular	Fungi: *Aspergillus* or mucormycosis *Nocardia*	Recurrent neoplasia
Diffuse	Viruses, e.g. CMV; *Chlamydia, Pneumocystis carinii, Toxoplasma gondii,* mycobacteria	Congestive cardiac failure, radiation pneumonitis, drug-induced lung injury, diffuse alveolar haemorrhage

This 30-year-old man was sent to the accident and emergency department by his GP. He was pyrexial and profoundly fatigued.

What is the likely underlying organism?

1. Group A *Streptococcus*
2. *Leptospira interrogans*
3. *Rickettsia conori*
4. *Borrelia burgdorferi*
5. *Mycoplasma*

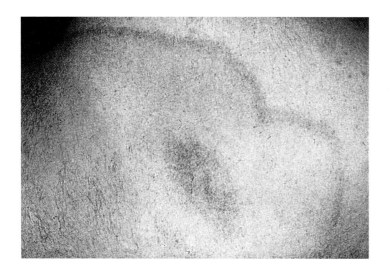

4. *Borrelia burgdorferi.*

The slide shows erythema chronicum migrans: the patient has contracted Lyme disease. The rash starts as a red macule at the site of the tick bite. It then spreads, typically with central clearing, to form annular erythemas. Constitutional symptoms may or may not be present at this stage.

Lyme disease is caused by the spirochaete *Borrelia burgdorferi*: transmission is by ticks of the *Ixodes* genus – *I. dammini* in the USA and *I. ricinus* in Europe – whose natural hosts include horses, deer and field mice.

- It is characterized by a progressive infectious course: infection originates at the site of the tick bite and the spirochaetes then disseminate haematogenously.
- Erythema chronicum migrans is the earliest feature in 70% of cases and one-third remember the initial tick bite. Fatigue, fever, headache and regional lymphadenopathy are well recognized.
- Fever is usual as the spirochaetes disseminate. Clinical features include:
  - *Skin*: cutaneous annular lesions, diffuse erythema and, with late untreated Lyme disease, acrodermatitis chronica atrophicans and lymphadenitis benigna cutis.
  - *Musculoskeletal*: arthralgia, myalgia, enthesopathy, chronic episodic arthritis affecting the large joints, typically the knee, with erosive changes occasionally occurring.
  - *Nervous system*: meningitis, radicular pain, cranial nerve palsies (a unilateral or bilateral VIIth nerve palsy is the commonest), mononeuritis multiplex, chronic encephalomyelitis, spastic paraparesis, cerebellar signs and dementia.
  - *Heart*: AV block, pancarditis.
  - *Other*: hepatitis, microscopic haematuria, conjunctivitis.
- The clinical diagnosis is supported by appropriate serology.

Treatment: Tetracyclines in adults for early disease and penicillin in children. Third-generation cephalosporins for late disease complications.

What is the diagnosis?

1. Klinefelter's syndrome
2. Hypothyroidism
3. Myotonic dystrophy
4. Kearns–Sayre syndrome
5. Acromegaly

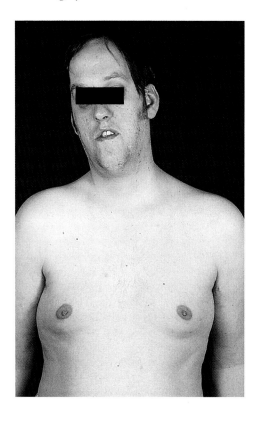

3. Myotonic dystrophy.

The typical facial appearances of frontal balding, expressionless forehead and myopathic facies are readily apparent. The patient also had bilateral ptosis hidden by the masking.

Myotonic dystrophy is the most common inherited neuromuscular disease in adults. It is an autosomal dominant disorder caused by a trinucleotide repeat expansion in the dystrophia myotonica protein kinase gene (DMPK), which is on chromosome 19. The repeat size typically increases with each generation and disease presentation therefore occurs earlier. This phenomenon is known as anticipation. The accumulation of mutant RNA transcripts in the nucleus is presumed to lead to the sequestration or activation of specific RNA binding proteins accounting for why a single gene defect can lead to such a diversity of features.

Clinical features include:

1. Wasting and weakness of the facial muscles, leading to bilateral ptosis and expressionless forehead; in the limbs, the forearm muscles are also particularly affected
2. Frontal balding
3. Cataracts
4. Gonadal atrophy
5. Cardiomyopathy
6. Oesophageal dysmotility
7. Impaired pulmonary ventilation
8. Low IQ.

This 10-year-old girl presented with a history of recurrent pyogenic infections and tender painful gums. She had a marked peripheral blood polymorphonuclear leukocytosis and normal lymphocyte count and immunoglobulin levels.

What is the most likely diagnosis?

1. Leukocyte adhesion molecule deficiency
2. Bruton's disease
3. Severe combined immunodeficiency
4. Scurvy
5. Diabetes mellitus

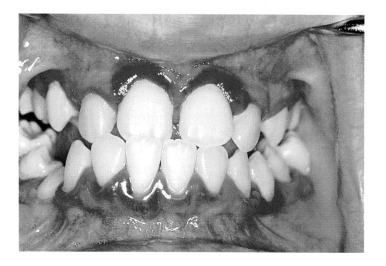

1. **Leukocyte adhesion molecule deficiency.**

The slide shows severe gum inflammation. The history of recurrent infections and sore gums, in concert with a leukocytosis, raises the possibility of leukocyte adhesion molecule deficiency.

Leukocyte adhesion deficiency is characterized by impaired neutrophil localization to tissues and impaired phagocytosis. Leukocyte adhesion deficiency type 1 is due to lack of CD18, the common β-chain of the integrins LFA-1, CR-3 and CR-4 used in cell migration and phagocytosis. Leukocyte adhesion deficiency type 2 is due to defective glycosylation, resulting in lack of ligands for E-selectin and P-selectin needed for migration.

Other phagocytic immunodeficiency states include:

- *Chédiak–Higashi syndrome* is a condition with impaired phagocyte response to chemoattractants and reduced killing of phagocytosed bacteria, due to a cytoskeletal defect.
- *Chronic granulomatous disease* is associated with increased infections due to catalase-positive organisms and leads to macrophage and granuloma formation at sites of infection. Chronic granulomatous disease is due to a defect of NADPH oxidase, leading to impaired oxygen-dependent killing.
- *Bruton's disease or X-linked agammaglobulinaemia* is characterized by low immunoglobulin levels and deficient antibody responses, but T-cell function and cell-mediated immunity to viral infections are normal.
- *Severe combined immunodeficiency* is a group of conditions with impaired cell-mediated immunity, leukopenia and low or absent antibody levels. Inheritance may be autosomal recessive due to adenosine deaminase deficiency or purine nucleoside phosphorylase deficiency. Other cases may be X-linked.

Note: Vitamin C deficiency (leading to scurvy) is a cause of gum hyperplasia and capillary fragility.

This patient was admitted through casualty with a cough and shortness of breath. Which of the following diagnoses can be *excluded* on the basis of the chest X-ray:

1. Extrinsic allergic alveolitis
2. Sarcoidosis
3. Berylliosis
4. Rheumatoid arthritis
5. Wegener's granulomatosis

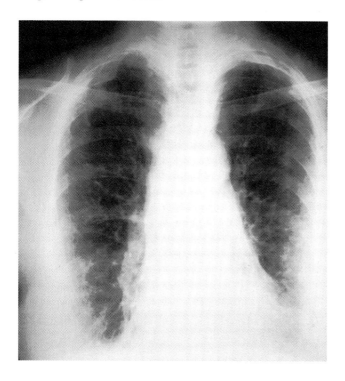

5. Wegener's granulomatosis.

The chest X-ray shows widespread interstitial shadowing and fibrotic change which is not consistent with a diagnosis of Wegener's granulomatosis.

The pulmonary manifestations of Wegener's granulomatosis include:
- Single or multiple nodules that may cavitate and heal with scar formation.
- Diffuse alveolar haemorrhages secondary to pulmonary capillaritis may present with haemoptysis and diffuse pulmonary infiltrates.
- Acute involvement of the trachea or bronchi can lead to inflammation, ulceration and malacia, leading to stenosis.
- In a small percentage of patients pleural effusions and hilar lymphadenopathy may develop.

The differential diagnosis of pulmonary fibrosis includes:
- Cryptogenic pulmonary fibrosis (idiopathic pulmonary fibrosis/usual interstitial pneumonitis): lower zones
- Pneumoconiosis:
  — Coalworker's: upper and mid zones
  — Silicosis: upper zones
  — Asbestosis: lower zones (holly leaf pleural plaques)
  — Berylliosis: upper zones
- Sarcoidosis: mid and upper
- Connective tissue diseases:
  — SLE: lower zones, diaphragms are often high
  — Scleroderma: lower zones
  — Rheumatoid arthritis: lower zones, nodules may be present
  — Ankylosing spondylitis: upper zones
- Chronic extrinsic allergic alveolitis, e.g. farmer's lung: upper zones
- Drugs, e.g.:
  — Amiodarone
  — Bleomycin
  — Busulfan
  — Melphalan
  — Cyclophosphamide
  — Nitrofurantoin.
- Tuberculosis: upper zones
- Bronchopulmonary aspergillosis: upper zones
- Previous irradiation: localized fibrosis.

Rare causes of fibrosis which are often associated with pronounced honeycombed change (and therefore preserving total lung volume) include:
- Neurofibromatosis
- Histiocytosis X
- Tuberose sclerosis
- Lymphangioleiomyomatosis

A 35-year-old woman with long-standing sarcoidosis is reviewed in outpatients. She has not felt well for the previous month and has a constant cough productive of brown sputum that has not responded to two courses of amoxycillin from her GP. The chest X-ray shown below was taken.

The most likely diagnosis is:

1. Tuberculosis
2. Bronchial carcinoma
3. Staphylococcal pneumonia
4. Aspergillosis
5. *Klebsiella* pneumonia

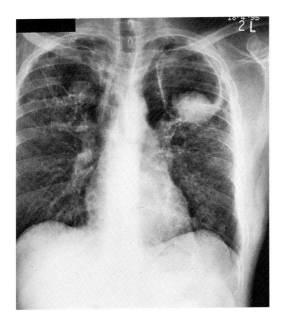

4. Aspergillosis.

The chest X-ray shows the classical appearance of aspergillomas in pre-formed cavities. This is a well-recognized complication of sarcoidosis. Sputum should be sent for *Aspergillus* culture and blood for *Aspergillus* precipitins.

CT scan will further define the extent of the fibrosis, degree of cavitations and number of aspergillomas.

Management will depend on the patient's clinical condition. Treatment options include oral itraconazole or a course of intravenous amphotericin.

If the patient presents with haemoptysis, angiography and embolization may be necessary if symptoms continue.

The development of a fungal ball in existing pulmonary cavities is most commonly associated with aspergilli, although other organisms including *Candida albicans* may produce this condition. In immunocompromised individuals aspergillosis may invade both the lung and extra pulmonary tissue; this is associated with a high mortality. In these cases intravenous amphotericin B is the recommended treatment.

What is the commonest respiratory complication of this syndrome?

1. Emphysema
2. Bronchiectasis
3. Cystic fibrosis
4. Bronchogenic carcinoma
5. Idiopathic pulmonary fibrosis

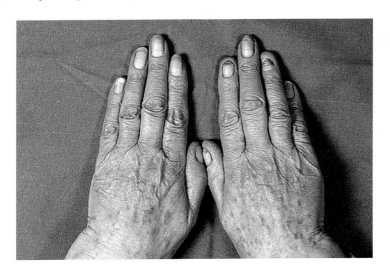

2. Bronchiectasis.

This patient has the yellow nail syndrome. The nails are smooth, thickened and over curved; the fingertips become uncovered because the nails are slow growing. The pathogenic mechanism appears to be an abnormality of lymphatic drainage.

The commonest respiratory complications are bronchiectasis and pleural effusions. **Bronchiectasis** describes chronic dilatation of one or more bronchi predisposing to chronic bacterial infection.

Causes of bronchiectasis include:
- *Immune deficiency*: panhypoglobulinaemia, selective immunoglobulin deficiency
- *Excessive immune response*: allergic bronchopulmonary aspergillosis
- *Mucociliary clearance defects*: Kartagener's syndrome (triad of sinusitis, situs inversus and bronchiectasis); cystic fibrosis; Young's syndrome (obstructive azoospermia and bronchiectasis)
- *Toxic insults*: aspiration of gastric contents
- *Mechanical obstruction*: intrinsic tumours and foreign bodies
- *Post-infective*: whooping-cough, persistent childhood infections, TB.

Other associations of the yellow nail syndrome include:
- Malignancy
- Hypothyroidism
- Hypogammaglobulinaemia
- Rheumatoid arthritis
- Others: AIDS, D-penicillamine therapy and nephritic syndrome.

A 35-year-old known intravenous drug abuser presents with a week's history of fevers and rigors.

a What is the likely underlying diagnosis?
1. Bacterial endocarditis
2. Streptococcal pneumonia
3. Miliary tuberculosis
4. *Pneumocystis carinii* pneumonia
5. Wegener's granulomatosis

b The two most important tests are:
1. Urine for pneumococcal antigen
2. Echocardiography
3. CT thorax
4. Sputum for acid-fast bacilli
5. Hepatic ultrasound
6. Blood cultures
7. HIV test
8. Hepatitis C serology
9. Hepatitis B serology
10. ANCA

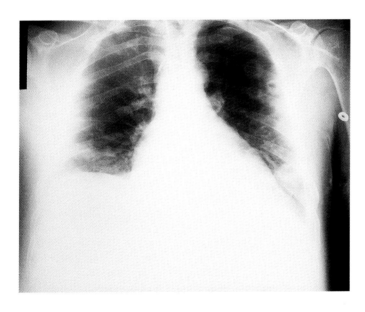

a 1. Bacterial endocarditis
b 2. Echocardiography and
  6. Blood cultures.

The slide shows two well-demarcated cavitating lesions.

Given the history of intravenous drug use associated with fevers and rigors, a strong possible diagnosis is right-sided endocarditis (most commonly due to *Staphylococcus aureus*). Valve vegetations can then lead to septic emboli lodging in the lungs and causing pulmonary infarction and consequent abscess formation.

The differential diagnosis of cavitating nodules on a chest X ray includes:

- Abscesses:
  — Post-aspiration (especially in unconscious patients following anaesthesia, excess alcohol consumption, epileptic fit, etc.)
  — Pneumonia, especially staphylococci or *Klebsiella*
- Neoplasia:
  — Primary or secondary tumours
- Tuberculosis:
  — Particularly upper lobes, often associated with calcification
- Pulmonary infarction;
  — Especially if caused by emboli from an infected valve (e.g. i.v. drug addicts) or venous lines (patients on chemotherapy or haemodialysis)
- Rheumatoid nodules
- Granulomas:
  — Wegener's granulomatosis
  — Sarcoid
- Fungal infections:
  — Histoplasmosis, coccidioidomycosis
- Bullae:
  — Commonly thin walled
- Pneumoconiosis or pulmonary fibrosis
- Cystic fibrosis
- Hydatid cysts.

Question 96

A 30-year female has become increasingly short of breath on minimal exertion. This had been associated with intermittent joint pain and stiffness over the last two years as well as some recent oral ulcers. Her echocardiogram is shown below.

What is the most likely underlying diagnosis?

1. Dilated cardiomyopathy
2. Atrial myxoma
3. Subacute bacterial endocarditis
4. Systemic lupus erythematosus
5. Mitral valve prolapse

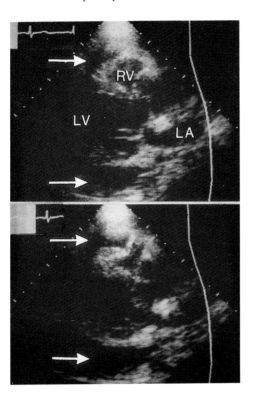

4. Systemic lupus erythematosus (SLE).

The slide shows a pericardial effusion with cardiac tamponade. This slide is a parasternal long-axis view and the pericardial effusion is of moderate size. Note that the two slides are during systole (top) and diastole (bottom). During diastole there is inward displacement of the right ventricular free wall, indicating that there is pericardial tamponade. This occurs when the pericardial pressure increases to a level that impedes ventricular filling.

Clinical signs of tamponade include: a sinus tachycardia, relative hypotension and pulsus paradoxus in excess of 10 mmHg, peripheral vasoconstriction, a raised jugular venous pressure that increases further with inspiration (Kussmaul's sign) and quiet heart sounds.

Urgent pericardiocentesis should be undertaken using the subcostal or apical route.

A pericarditis with or without an effusion is the most frequent cardiac complication of SLE. Others include: myocarditis, cardiomyopathy that can also affect the conducting system, myocardial infarction secondary to both coronary arteritis and an increased incidence of atherosclerosis, endocardial involvement inducing thromboembolism and infective or non-infective (Libman–Sacks endocarditis).

Causes of idiopathic pericarditis
- Infections:
  - Viral
  - Bacterial – including TB, syphilis
  - Mycotic: histoplasmosis, actinomycosis, nocardia
  - Amoebiasis
- Post cardiac injury:
  - Cardiotomy
  - Myocardial infarction and Dressler's syndrome
  - Radiotherapy
  - Trauma
  - Aortic dissection
- In association with systemic disease:
  - Connective tissue disorders: (RA, SLE, systemic sclerosis, rheumatic fever, Churg–Strauss, Giant cell arteritis)
  - Uraemia
  - Hypothyroidism
  - Sarcoidosis
  - Familial Mediterranean fever
- Secondary to neoplasia:
  - Either primary or secondary
- Drug-induced:
  - Procainamide, hydralazine.

What is the clinical diagnosis?

1. Subacute bacterial endocarditis
2. Marantic endocarditis
3. Libman–Sacks endocarditis
4. Atrial myxoma
5. Mitral stenosis

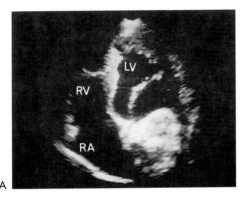

A

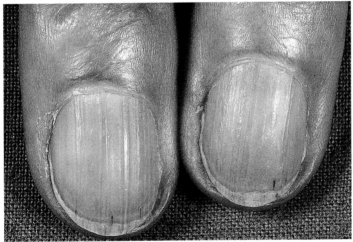

B

4. Atrial myxoma.

- *Slide A*: an apical four-chamber view of the heart, showing a large echogenic mass filling the left atrium (LV, left ventricle; M, myxoma; RA, right atrium; RV, right ventricle)
- *Slide B*: demonstrates the typical appearance of splinter haemorrhages.

Atrial myxomas are lobulated gelatinous masses that are the commonest primary cardiac neoplasm occurring most commonly in the left atrium.

They are more common in females than in males. Three-quarters arise from the fossa ovalis and are in the left atrium; the rest occur in the right atrium, apart from very rare ventricular lesions. Macroscopically, myxomas are pedunculated and covered in adherent thrombus.

Their presentation may mimic that of other more common systemic diseases.

Important clinical presentations include:

Symptoms and signs of left atrial outflow obstruction	As a differential diagnosis of mitral stenosis • The presenting symptoms therefore include progressive breathlessness, orthopnoea, paroxysmal nocturnal dyspnoea and atrial arrhythmias
Systemic embolization	Often occurring when the patient is in sinus rhythm
As pyrexia of unknown origin	Features include: weight loss, Raynaud's, finger clubbing, abnormal serum proteins with elevated immunoglobulin levels Other haematological findings include elevated ESR, a normochromic normocytic anaemia, leukocytosis and thrombocytosis. There may be evidence of haemolysis • Initial differential diagnoses include infective endocarditis and occult malignancy
Cardiovascular signs	These are usually non-specific. Classically, signs including mitral systolic and diastolic murmurs change with posture. Rarely a tumour 'plop' may be heard in early diastole

Echocardiography is the investigation of choice. Once the diagnosis is confirmed, urgent full-thickness surgical excision is indicated. Regular echocardiographic follow-up is indicated, as the rate of recurrence is up to 5% of cases.

This is the peripheral blood film from a patient with a left radial nerve palsy.

a What does the blood film show?
1. Helmut cells
2. Smear cells
3. A macrocytosis
4. Basophilic stippling
5. Acanthocytes

b What is the underlying diagnosis?
1. B$_{12}$/folate deficiency
2. Myelofibrosis
3. Amyloidosis
4. Hypothyroidism
5. Lead poisoning

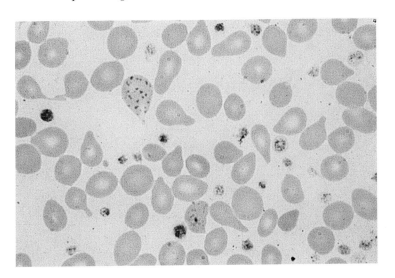

a 4. Basophilic stippling
b 5. Lead poisoning.

The peripheral red blood cells show basophilic stippling. The coarse (punctate) dots represent condensed RNA in the cytoplasm. In the context of a radial nerve palsy the most likely diagnosis is lead poisoning. Basophilic stippling does not reflect the severity of the poisoning; it may be absent altogether in severe cases.

Basophilic stippling is also seen in other disorders of haemoglobin synthesis such as pyrimidine-5-nucleotidase deficiency, acquired sideroblastic anaemia and homozygous beta-thalassaemias.

Which of the following is *not* associated with the deformities shown in this slide?

1. Charcot–Marie–Tooth disease (hereditary motor and sensory neuropathy)
2. Old polio infection
3. Friedreich's ataxia
4. Spina bifida
5. Dystrophia myotonica

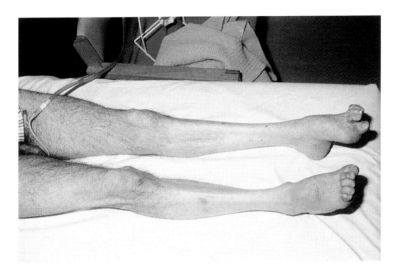

5. Dystrophia myotonica.

The abnormalities shown on the slide are:

- Distal muscle wasting which stops around mid thigh. This has been described as the 'inverted champagne bottles' type of appearance.
- Clawed toes and a pes cavus deformity.

The differential diagnosis of pes cavus and muscle wasting includes:

Charcot–Marie–Tooth disease Peroneal muscular atrophy/hereditary motor and sensory neuropathy (HMSN)*	• A hereditary motor and sensory neuropathy • Clinical features include a 'high-stepping' gait due to bilateral foot drop; wasting of the small muscles of the hand; thickened peripheral nerves; areflexia; distal sensory neuropathy; digital trophic ulceration; upper limb tremor; and scoliosis • Autosomal dominant with variable penetrance
Old polio infection	• Generally presents with asymmetrical lower motor neurone weakness and reduced or absent reflexes. Can develop a progressive wasting disease
Friedreich's ataxia	• A hereditary spinocerebellar degenerative disease • High-arched palate/kyphoscoliosis/bilateral pes cavus • Cerebellar signs: ataxia, dysarthria, nystagmus • Dorsal column loss: impaired vibration and position sense • Other features include peripheral neuropathy, corticospinal tract involvement; extensor plantar responses, optic atrophy, cardiomyopathy, diabetes • Autosomal recessive, occasionally autosomal dominant inheritance
Spina bifida	• Incomplete closure of the bony vertebral canal, usually in the lumbrosacral region • There can be a lipoma, sinus, dimple or hypertrichosis over the defect • Typically asymmetrical shortening with distal wasting and associated deformity, sensory loss and a neuropathic bladder

*Two types of peroneal muscular atrophy may be distinguished. Type I is commoner, has an earlier age of onset (first decade) and is associated with more severe clinical features than type II. Peripheral nerve thickening, diffuse demyelination and reduced nerve conduction velocities are features of type I and not type II.

What is the diagnosis?

1. Dilated cardiomyopathy
2. Constrictive cardiomyopathy
3. Atrial myxoma
4. Hypertrophic obstructive cardiomyopathy (HOCM)
5. Mitral stenosis

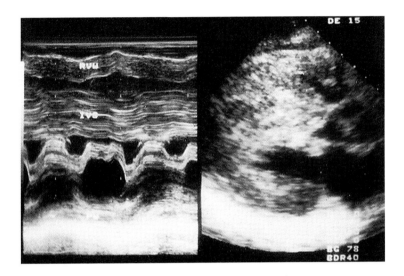

4. Hypertrophic obstructive cardiomyopathy (HOCM).

This slide shows a parasternal long-axis view (right) and the M mode recording (left) from a patient with HOCM. There is disproportional (asymmetric) septal hypertrophy (3–4 cm), poor systolic thickening of the septum and a systolic anterior motion of the mitral valve (SAM). Note also that the right ventricular wall is hypertrophied. IVS, intraventricular septum; RVW, right ventricular wall.

HOCM is inherited as an autosomal dominant trait, although sporadic cases occur.

- It often presents in the second decade with shortness of breath resulting from an elevated left atrial pressure.
- Other presentations include syncope, angina and palpitations (atrial and ventricular arrhythmias are common).
- Clinical signs include:
  — A jerky but sustained pulse with a rapid initial upstroke followed by a sustained component
  — A double apical impulse composed of a palpable atrial beat followed by the prominent left ventricular impulse
  — IIIrd and IVth heart sounds
  — A late systolic apical murmur whose intensity is diminished by squatting or isometric hand exercises and increased by amyl nitrate or the Valsalva manoeuvre.

Currently the detection and treatment of ventricular arrhythmias appear to provide the best approach to reducing the risk of sudden death. Amiodarone is the drug of choice for arrhythmia prophylaxis.

This patient presented to her GP with malaise, fever and exertional shortness of breath.
    What is the likely diagnosis?

1. Sarcoidosis
2. *Mycoplasma* pneumonia
3. Mitral stenosis
4. Variegate porphyria
5. Systemic lupus erythematosus

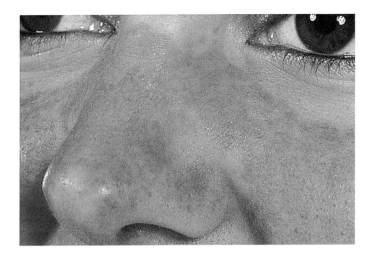

5. **Systemic lupus erythematosus (SLE).**

The slide shows the typical photosensitive rash of SLE.

SLE is associated with many mucocutaneous features. The most characteristic are the photosensitive malar rash and discoid lupus. Subacute cutaneous lupus produces a generalized non-scarring rash which is either psoriasiform or annular.

Other dermatological features include:

Bullous lesions, urticaria, angio-oedematous areas, a small-vessel vasculitis, livedo reticularis (anti-phospholipid antibody-positive or cryoglobulin-associated), lupus profundus (inflammation of subcutaneous fat), Raynaud's phenomenon.

See page 239 Appendix 1 for table of features.

This 45-year-old woman presented with cold blue left second and third fingers. A digital angiogram was performed what is the diagnosis?

1. Takayasu's arteritis
2. Peripheral emboli
3. Buerger's disease
4. Syphilis
5. Giant cell arteritis

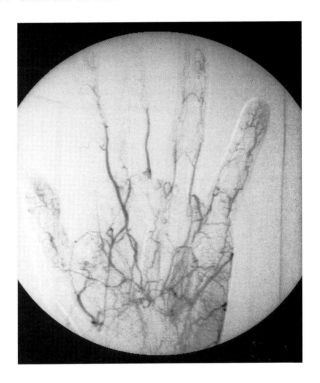

3. Buerger's disease.

The angiogram is typical of Buerger's disease (thromboangiitis obliterans) with loss of the digital arteries and typical corkscrew collaterals.

Thromboangiitis obliterans is an inflammatory occlusive peripheral vascular disease of unknown aetiology that affects medium-sized arteries and veins. It occurs more commonly in males and almost exclusively in smokers.

The clinical features of thomboangiitis obliterans include a triad of claudication, Raynaud's phenomenon and a migratory superficial vein thrombophlebitis.

- Claudication most commonly in the calves, feet, forearms and hands, reflecting the distal distribution of disease
- Gangrene at the fingertips due to digital ischaemia can occur
- Brachial and popliteal pulses are present but radial, ulnar and tibial pulse can be absent.

There is no specific treatment except abstention from tobacco. Vascular perfusion improves when individuals are no longer exposed to cigarettes. With acute ischaemia intravenous prostacyclin and oral aspirin may help.

This 35-year-old patient presented with a fractured right femur. What is the diagnosis?

1. Cushing's disease
2. Osteogenesis imperfecta
3. Ehlers–Danlos syndrome
4. Marfan's disease
5. Scleromalacia perforans

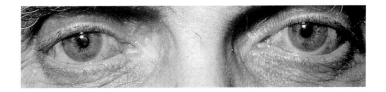

2. Osteogenesis imperfecta.

The combination of blue sclerae and fracture suggests osteogenesis imperfecta.

The differential diagnosis of blue sclerae is:

1. Osteogenesis imperfecta
2. Pseudoxanthoma elasticum
3. Ehlers–Danlos syndrome
4. Marfan's disease
5. Hyperthyroidism.

Osteogenesis imperfecta (OI) is caused by mutations of the type I collagen gene. Type I collagen is the main collagen component of bone, and consists of a triple helix (α_1 and α_2 chains). Type I OI is mild, and patients present with blue sclerae, deafness and fractures. Type II OI is the severe infantile form resulting in early death, type III shows short stature due to long bone deformity, grey sclera and ligamentous laxity, while type IV demonstrates variable bone fragility and normal sclera. Types I and IV are inherited in an autosomal dominant fashion, while types II and III are autosomal recessive or sporadic. Treatment is not satisfactory, but maintaining muscle tone with exercise and using orthopaedic devices to prevent deformity and scoliosis are useful.

Other notes: Ehlers–Danlos disease consists of 10 different types, with autosomal dominant, recessive and X-linked recessive inheritance. The abnormalities are in the structure of types I and III collagen.

The clinical features vary and include the following:

- The skin is thin and inelastic and heals poorly, leading to scarring and 'fish mouth wounds'
- The joints are hypermobile and patients are prone to recurrent dislocations
- Visceral and arterial rupture is found particularly in type IV
- Ocular lesions include scleral tears, keratoconus and occasionally angioid streaks.

This 25-year-old woman presented to the casualty department complaining of ankle pain.

What is the single most important investigation to perform?

1. FBC
2. Blood cultures
3. CRP
4. Chest X-ray
5. ASO titre

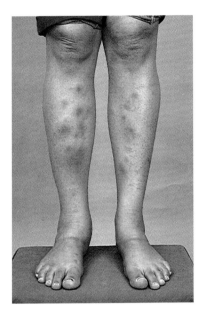

4. Chest X-ray.

This is the classical appearance of **erythema nodosum**.

- It classically presents with crops of raised red tender lesions over the shins, though they can occur on any fat-covered area of the body.
- Acute lesions evolve over a 10-day period into blue-violet covered areas that gradually fade.
- Histologically a panniculitis with a perivascular mixed cell infiltrate is seen on biopsy.
- Patients may be systemically unwell with malaise, fever, arthralgia or arthritis, often most marked in the knees and ankles.

A chest X-ray would be the single most important test to exclude pulmonary tuberculosis and look for evidence of bilateral hilar lymphadenopathy, which would suggest a diagnosis of sarcoidosis (Lofgren's syndrome).

Erythema nodosum is idiopathic in the majority of cases but well-recognized associations include:

- Infections:
  - Streptococcal
  - *Yersinia*
  - Tuberculosis
  - Psittacosis
  - Deep fungal infections
  - Cat-scratch fever
  - Lymphogranuloma venerum
- Sarcoidosis
- Drugs:
  - Oral contraceptive pill
  - Sulfonamides
  - Barbiturates
  - Salicylates
- Inflammatory bowel disease:
  - Crohn's disease and ulcerative colitis
- Behçet's disease
- Malignancies:
  - Lymphoma and leukaemia.

Many patients require non-steroidal anti-inflammatory drugs initially to control their symptoms.

This man presented with interscapular pain.

a What does the echocardiogram show?
 1. Ventricular septal rupture
 2. Aortic dissection
 3. Pericardial tamponade
 4. Papillary muscle rupture
 5. Left ventricular aneurysm rupture

b List three of the following that are considered to be predisposing factors in causing this:
 1. Hypertension
 2. Coarctation of the aorta
 3. Marfan's syndrome
 4. Secondary syphilis
 5. Myocardial infarction

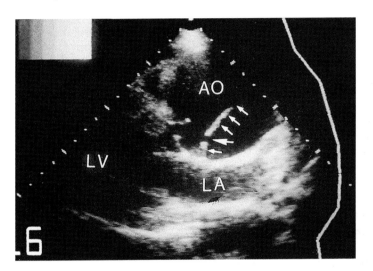

a 2. Aortic dissection
b 1. Hypertension; 2. coarctation of the aorta; 3. Marfan's syndrome.

The slide shows a parasternal long-axis view from a patient with an aortic dissection. Note the dilated (7 cm) ascending aorta with a posteriorly situated intimal flap (arrows). (AO, ascending aorta; LA, left atrium; LV, left ventricle).

- The thoracic aorta is the commonest site for dissecting aneurysms. The dissection usually starts in the ascending aorta and extends to involve the arch, descending and abdominal aorta. Extension of the dissection may result in limb ischaemia, spinal artery occlusion, mesenteric infarction and renal failure. Dissecting aneurysms commonly occur in men aged between 40 and 70 years; predisposing factors include hypertension, coarctation of the aorta and Marfan's syndrome. Tearing interscapular pain is the commonest presenting symptom, with pain radiating into the neck and arms. Other presenting complaints include pleuritic chest pain, cardiac pain (as the dissection occludes a coronary ostium), syncope and dyspnoea. Clinical signs include an aortic diastolic murmur, a pericardial friction rub and a difference in blood pressure or radial pulse between the right and left arms.
- The chest X-ray may show widening of the upper mediastinum but this is unreliable. The diagnosis, if suspected, should be confirmed using echocardiography, contrast-enhanced CT scanning or MR imaging.
- Immediate management of a thoracic aortic dissection involves pain relief and control of blood pressure, followed by surgical repair of the aorta. Overall, 50% of patients die within five days and 90% within six months.

Other notes: Patients with syphilitic aortitis may be asymptomatic. Recognized manifestations include saccular aneurysms in the ascending aorta (asymptomatic or symptomatic pain; pressure on adjacent structures may lead to SVC obstruction, hoarseness etc. and rupture), aortic regurgitation and myocardial ischaemia due to coronary ostial stensosis.

The urine microscopy of this patient showed red blood cells and several red cell casts per high-powered field.

What is the diagnosis?

1. Relapsing polychondritis
2. Congenital syphilis
3. Wegener's granulomatosis
4. Lepromatous leprosy
5. Paget's disease

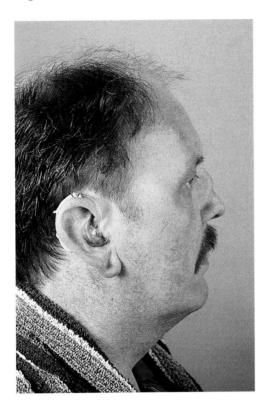

3. **Wegener's granulomatosis.**

The urine sediment indicates glomerulonephritis; combined with upper respiratory tract disease (collapse of the nasal bridge and hearing loss) this strongly suggests a diagnosis of **Wegener's granulomatosis**. This is a small-vessel vasculitis which most commonly involves: the upper respiratory tract (involvement of nose, sinuses, ears), the lower respiratory tract (nodular and cavitating lesions) and the kidney (focal necrotizing (crescenteric) glomerulonephritis). Evidence of disease in two or more of these sites with histology showing a small-vessel necrotizing vasculitis, with associated granuloma formation, confirms the diagnosis. Anti-neutrophil cytoplasmic antibodies (ANCA) are sensitive serological markers for Wegener's granulomatosis and microscopic polyarteritis nodosa (a related small-vessel vasculitic illness: systemic symptoms, lower respiratory and renal disease manifestations). Patients with Wegener's are usually C-ANCA positive, the antibodies being directed against proteinase-3. Other clinical features of Wegener's granulomatosis include: fever and malaise; polyarthralgia; a vasculitic rash; scleritis, uveitis and proptosis; pericarditis, myocarditis and arrhythmias; mononeuritis multiplex and intracerebral granulomas.

Before effective treatment was available, 80% of patients with Wegener's granulomatosis died within one year, and the mean survival was five months. Since the introduction of cyclophosphamide combined with corticosteroids, remission rates are in excess of 90%. Plasma exchange has proved beneficial for those patients with a rapidly progressive glomerulonephritis or lung haemorrhage.

The differential diagnosis of a collapsed nasal bridge with intact overlying skin includes:

1. Wegener's granulomatosis
2. Relapsing polychondritis
3. Congenital syphilis
4. Trauma.

This 25-year-old actor presented to rheumatology outpatients with a
swollen right knee and a painful left third toe.

What is the diagnosis?

1. Behçet's syndrome
2. Reiter's syndrome
3. Gonorrhoea
4. Secondary syphilis
5. Systemic lupus erythematosus

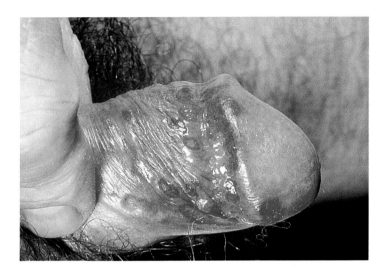

2. Reiter's syndrome.

This is the typical appearance of circinate balanitis. Painless vesicles first appear on the coronal margin of the prepuce and adjacent glans; they can rupture to form superficial erosions that may coalesce to form the typical circinate pattern.

Combined with the history this suggests an underlying diagnosis of **Reiter's syndrome**. This is a triad of synovitis, urethritis and conjunctivitis.

Two distinct types of reactive arthritis are recognized:

1. Complicating urethral tract infections. Most often sexually acquired. *Chlamydia* is the underlying organism in 60% of cases.
2. Following episodes of dysentery with *Salmonella*, *Shigella*, *Yersinia* and *Campylobacter*.

- It is typically seen in patients between the ages of 16 and 35 years.
- Post-venereal reactive arthritis is much commoner in males than females and there is a strong genetic association with HLA B27.
- Recurrent or chronic disease occurs in up to 60% of patients.

Clinical features include:

Musculoskeletal	Oligoarthritis	Typically affecting the large joints of the lower limbs, although upper limb involvement is also described
	Enthesopathy	Inflammation of tendon insertions, particularly the Achilles, and plantar fasciitis
	Sacroiliitis	
Ocular	Conjunctivitis	
	Iritis	
Cutaneous	Circinate balanitis	Affects 20–50%
	Keratoderma blennorrhagicum	Yellow, waxy, warty lesions on the soles of the feet occur in up to 15% of patients
	Painless oral ulceration	Occurs in up to 10% of patients
	Nail dystrophy	
Systemic symptoms	Malaise and fever	Other rare features include: cardiac conduction defects, aortic regurgitation, pericarditis, pulmonary infiltrates and peripheral neuropathy

This patient presented with severe back pain. A T1-weighted MRI scan was performed.

What is the underlying diagnosis?

1. Multiple myeloma
2. Cushing's syndrome
3. Tuberculous osteomyelitis
4. Metastatic disease
5. Hyperthyroidism

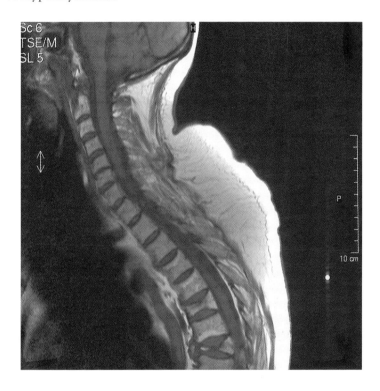

2. Cushing's syndrome.

The most prominent feature on sagittal magnetic resonance T1-weighted image is the presence of a large supraclavicular fat pad (buffalo hump), consistent with a diagnosis of Cushing's syndrome. This has led to osteoporosis and osteoporotic collapse of the 7th and 9th thoracic vertebrae.

- Clinical symptoms of Cushing's syndrome include weight gain, menstrual irregularity and amenorrhoea, hirsuitism; impotence in the male, depression, muscle weakness and fractures secondary to osteoporosis.
- Characteristic signs include hypertension, tissue wasting, abdominal striae, water retention and abnormal fat distribution – supraclavicular fat pads are well recognized. A proximal myopathy is commonly present.

A 35-year-old doctor presents with a six-month history of a painful swollen wrist.

He is otherwise systemically well and his inflammatory markers (ESR and CRP) are normal. Aspiration was performed on two occasions; no organisms were seen on Gram or Ziehl–Neelsen staining and the wrist was injected with corticosteroids. The pain and swelling have increased and a biopsy has been performed – the histology is shown.

The most likely diagnosis is:

1. Sarcoidosis
2. Rheumatoid arthritis
3. Tuberculosis
4. Gonococcal arthritis
5. Haemachromatosis

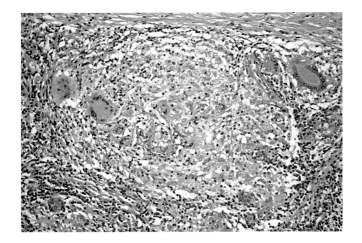

3. Tuberculosis.

The biopsy shows a caseating granulomatous infiltrate. This is typical of tuberculosis. Acid-fast bacilli were seen on Ziehl–Neelsen stain.

Synovial biopsy and culture are imperative in patients presenting with a chronic monoarthritis in the absence of a firm diagnosis.

- Tuberculosis in the appendicular skeleton often presents with a chronic monoarthritis with little systemic upset. Only 50% can be shown to have other organ involvement, the lungs being most commonly affected.
- Tuberculosis of the spine usually involves the thoracic spine, starting in the anterior body of a vertebra before spreading to the intervertebral disc. Malignant processes, in contrast, spare the intervertebral disc.
- This patient should be treated with combination anti-tuberculous therapy for at least 12 months.

What is the diagnosis?

1. Tuberculosis
2. Wegener's granulomatosis
3. Lymphoma
4. Sarcoidosis
5. Multicentric reticulohistiocytosis

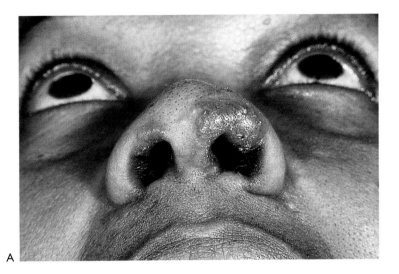

A

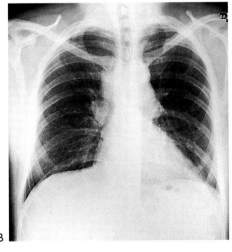

B

4. Sarcoidosis.

The typical red nodular lesions of lupus pernio are well seen; the chest X-ray shows bilateral hilar lymphadenopathy.

The lesions of lupus pernio are disfiguring; they occur more commonly in women and are much more florid in blacks than whites. Lupus pernio is particularly associated with sarcoidosis affecting the upper respiratory tract and overall is associated with the chronic fibrotic type of sarcoid.

The cutaneous manifestations of **sarcoidosis** are many and varied and include:

- Erythema nodosum
- Papulonodular sarcoid: smooth red-brown lesions, which can occur anywhere on the body
- Annular sarcoid and scar sarcoid.

The pathological finding in sarcoidosis is the non-necrotizing granuloma, although this is not specific for sarcoid. Other conditions that may be confused are tuberculosis and deep-seated fungal infections, although these usually have frank necrosis. Malignant diseases can also cause a granulomatous reaction, lymphoma being the commonest.

Other investigations, which may be helpful, are:

- Serum ACE levels (elevated in 70% of patients), hypercalcaemia and hypercalcuria
- CT imaging, which can confirm hilar lymphadenopathy, demonstrate fibrosis and show characteristic beading of the bronchovascular bundles
- Gallium scans, which demonstrate increased uptake in involved sites
- Bronchoalveolar lavage showing a lymphocytosis (CD4:CD8 >3.5).

Note: Multicentric reticulohistiocytosis is a rare disease affecting skin and joints. Firm yellow-red papules occur on the face, hands and torso. Biopsy demonstrates multinucleated giant cells; the arthritis is a symmetrical destructive polyarthritis affecting the hands and cervical spine.

This 58-year-old female presented with bilateral ankle pain and a rash of two weeks' duration. Urine showed protein++, blood+. Liver function tests AST 65, ALT 76, normal alkaline phosphatase and normal bilirubin.

Which of the following complement profiles would you expect?

1. Low C3, normal C4 and low CH50
2. Low C3, low C4 and low CH50
3. Normal C3, normal C4 and low CH50
4. Normal C3, low C4 and low CH50
5. Normal C3, low C4 and normal CH50

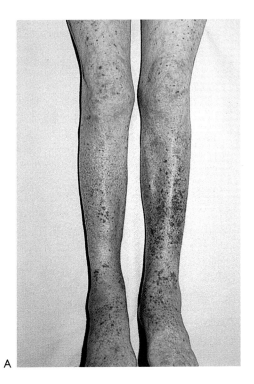

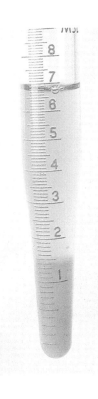

A

B

4. Normal C3, low C4 and low CH50.

Slide A shows an extensive purpuric rash and slide B shows an unspun cryoprecipitate. This lady has mixed cryoglobulinaemia, presenting with a vasculitic rash, arthritis and glomerulonephritis.

Cryoglobulinaemia is an immune complex-mediated vasculitis. There are three types:

- *Type I*: the cryoprecipitate is composed of a single monoclonal immunoglobulin without any antibody activity. This can be found in patients with multiple myeloma, Waldenström's macroglobulinaemia or idiopathic monoclonal gammopathy.
- *Types II and III* are mixed cryoglobulinaemias: they are composed of at least two immunoglobulins. In type II they are composed of monoclonal immunoglobulin (usually monoclonal immunoglobulin with rheumatoid activity to IgG). In type III all the components are polyclonal.

Mixed cryoglobulinaemias account for the majority (60–70%). Many cases with type II cryoglobulins were initially labelled as essential cryoglobulinaemia because no underlying cause could be found. It has now been found that many of these patients have underlying hepatitis C infection. (This would account for this lady's transaminitis.) The typical complement profile is one of a normal C3, low C4 and low CH50.

Other causes of types II and III cryoglobulinaemia include connective tissue diseases, leukaemia, hepatobiliary diseases, infectious diseases and post-infectious glomerulonephritis.

Mixed cryoglobulins affect females in particular and present most commonly with a triad of skin renal, and joint disease:

- *Skin*: cutaneous vasculitis is seen in virtually all patients with prominent lower limb purpura, often progressing to frank ulceration.
- *Renal*: renal disease due to membranoproliferative glomerulonephritis with immunoglobulin and complement deposition occurs in up to 50% of all patients with mixed cryoglobulinaemia and almost exclusively with type II. Nephrotic syndrome and hypertension are common sequelae.
- *Joints*: symmetrical arthralgia affecting the hands, knees and elbows is common in mixed cryoglobulinaemia but rarely progresses to frank arthritis.

Alpha-interferon combined with ribavirin is effective in reducing cryoglobulin levels in patients with hepatitis C and concomitant cryoglobulinaemia. Patients with underlying renal disease presenting with a rash and arthritis have a worse prognosis and are more likely to benefit from plasma exchange, high-dose corticosteroids and cyclophosphamide.

What is the clinical diagnosis?

1. Keloid
2. Morphea
3. Lupus vulgaris
4. Bowen's disease
5. Necrobiosis lipoidica

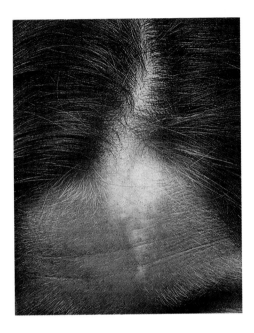

2. Morphea.

The slide shows the typical appearance of morphea or linear scleroderma and this describes localized sclerosis of the skin. Sometimes this midline facial distribution has also been given the term 'coup de sabre'. This pattern tends to occur more commonly in children and can be associated with an underlying defect in skull growth.

Morphea and other localized patterns of skin sclerosis usually present in isolation of other features seen with systemic sclerosis.

The scleroderma spectrum of disorders encompasses a number of diseases which tend to have skin sclerosis and Raynaud's phenomenon in common:

- *Limited cutaneous systemic sclerosis* (formerly termed CREST (**c**alcinosis, **R**aynaud's, o**e**sophagus, **s**cleroderma and **t**elangectasia): this is the most common, accounting for over 60% of cases. The typical patient is female between the ages of 30 and 50 and has had Raynaud's phenomenon for a long time. She then develops sclerodermatous skin changes in (i) the hands, which do not progress above the elbows, (ii) feet, which do not progress above the knees, and (iii) face and neck. 90% of patients are ANA+ and 70% anti-centromere antibody+.
- *Diffuse cutaneous systemic sclerosis*: this usually presents acutely. There may be widespread painful swelling of the extremities and face, associated with pruritus, rapid weight loss and general symptoms of fatigue. Subsequently the skin becomes tight and thickened proximal to the elbows, with involvement of the truncal areas. Systemic complications include arthralgia/arthritis, pulmonary fibrosis, oesophageal hypomobility, bacterial overgrowth with malabsorption, pseudo-obstruction, myopathy, cardiomyopathy and pericardial effusions, scleroderma and renal hypertensive crisis. 90% of patients are ANA+ and 40% anti-Scl (anti-topoisomerase)+.
- *Scleroderma sine scleroderma*: describes a rare group of patients (<2%) who present without the skin changes of scleroderma but have all the systemic complications.
- *Overlap syndromes*: (sometimes also termed 'mixed connective tissue disease' or 'undifferentiated connective tissue syndrome') describe patients who have features of other connective tissue diseases.

This female was referred to outpatients by her GP. Her blood pressure was 160/95 mmHg.

Which one of the following tests would be most helpful in forwarding the diagnosis?

1. Plasma ACTH level
2. Metapyrone suppression test
3. 24-hour urinary free cortisol
4. Antibodies against ds DNA
5. Renal ultrasound

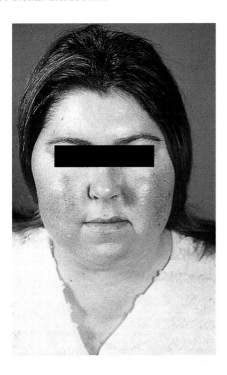

3. 24-hour urinary free cortisol.
The slide shows the typical Cushingoid appearance with moon face and plethora. Other features of Cushing's syndrome include: truncal obesity, hirsutism, easy bruising, osteoporosis, proximal myopathy, hypertension, diabetes and depressive psychosis.

Cushing's syndrome is defined as the signs and symptoms of excess circulating levels of cortisol

Differential diagnosis of Cushing's syndrome
- Iatrogenic: exogenous glucocorticoids
- Non-iatrogenic:
  — ACTH dependent:
  1. Cushing's disease (80%): pituitary-dependent bilateral adrenal hyperplasia, often the result of a basophil microadenoma
  2. Ectopic ACTH from a benign or malignant tumour (5–10%), e.g. oat cell carcinoma, pancreatic tumour. In these cases patients often have a hypokalaemic metabolic alkalosis and hypertension, increased skin pigmentation, muscle weakness and diabetes dominate the clinical picture.
  — ACTH independent:
  1. Primary adrenal adenoma (5–10%)
  2. Primary adrenal carcinoma – rare; often associated with virilization
  3. Micronodular adrenal dysplasia
  4. Pseudo-Cushing's syndrome due to alcohol abuse or associated with a severe depressive psychosis.

The investigations of suspected Cushing's syndrome fall into two parts:
1. Confirm cortisol excess:
   — raised 24-hour urine free cortisol
   — Failure of cortisol levels to suppress following administration of low-dose dexamethasone (0.5 mg dexamethasone 6-hourly for 24 hours). *Note:* Stress, pregnancy and the oral contraceptive may all raise the midnight cortisol and 24-hour excretion. Patients with pseudo-Cushing's should suppress; patients with true Cushing's should not. Some normal, obese, depressed or alcoholic patients suppress poorly; patients with cyclical Cushing's may suppress normally.
2. Determining the cause:
   — Plasma ACTH levels, very high with ectopic ACTH, raised in Cushing's disease and undetectable with adrenal carcinoma or adenoma
   — High-dose dexamethasone suppression test suppresses ACTH and plasma cortisol in Cushing's disease
   — Metyrapone test: metyrapone inhibits 11-beta-hydroxylase and therefore cortisol synthesis and will cause a further rise in ACTH and thus 17-oxogenic steroids in Cushing's disease but not with ectopic ACTH
   — MRI of the pituitary and CT of the adrenals. Selenium-75 cholesterol scans for adrenal adenomas. Arteriography and venography to localize the exact source of ACTH.

a What is the diagnosis?
  1. Discoid eczema
  2. Psoriasis
  3. Erythema nodosum
  4. Pityriasis rosea
  5. Lichen planus

b Which of the following drugs could have exacerbated this skin condition?
  1. Lithium
  2. Amoxycillin
  3. Aspirin
  4. Ibuprofen
  5. Metronidazole

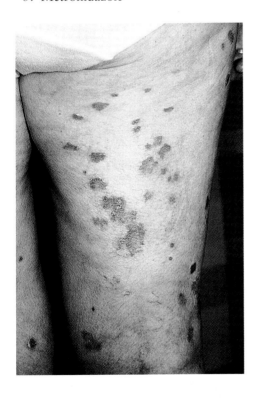

a 2. Psoriasis
b 1. Lithium.

The slide shows well-demarcated dull red plaques with overlying silvery scales that are typical of psoriasis.

A number of medications can exacerbate psoriasis. These include antimalarials, lithium, beta-blockers, alcohol and tobacco. Other precipitants include HIV and streptococcal infections.

Psoriasis is a common inflammatory hyperproliferative skin condition that is often inherited and sometimes associated with disorders of the joints and nails. There are a number of morphological variations and psoriasis has a predilection for a number of different sites, particularly the scalp and the extensor areas.

Type	Clinical features	Treatment
Plaque psoriasis	The most common lesions are well demarcated and range from a few millimetres to several centimetres in diameter. They are pink or red with large, dry, silvery-white polygonal scales (like candle grease). Elbows, knees lower back and scalp are the commonest sites	Vitamin D analogues Local retinoids Local steroids Dithranol Coal tar *If extensive:* UVB PUVA Methotrexate
Guttate psoriasis	Usually seen in adolescents and young adults. Characterized by crops of small drop-like papules and plaques. Often found in association with strep. sore throat infections	Systemic antibiotics Weak tar preparations Mild local steroid
Pustular psoriasis	Fine superficial pustules, often with fine desquamation, occur on the palm and soles	Mod. potent local steroid Local retinoid
Erythrodermic psoriasis	Rare. Can be provoked by the withdrawal of steroids or by a drug eruption. The skin is uniformly red with variable scaling.	Inpatient treatment with ichthammol paste Methotrexate, cyclosporin may be required.

Note: Pityriasis rosea may be confused with guttate psoriasis but lesions tend to be oval rather than round and run along the rib line. A herald plaque may precede the rash and lesions are usually confined to the upper trunk.

This female presented to the accident and emergency department with abdominal pain.

Which of the following would confirm the diagnosis?

1. Measurement of ACTH levels
2. Barium swallow
3. Short synacthen test
4. Renal and adrenal ultrasound
5. Renal biopsy

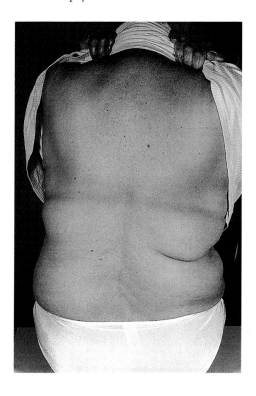

3. Short synacthen test.

The slide shows hyperpigmentation around the pressure areas of this lady's bra straps. This is the typical hyperpigmentation seen with **Addison's disease** (primary adrenal failure associated with increased levels of ACTH and beta-MSH).

Pigmentation may also be seen: in mucosal areas such as the buccal mucosa, in the palmar creases, in areas of skin exposed to light and in scars acquired after the onset of Addison's disease.

Abdominal pain is a typical presenting feature of Addison's disease. Other clinical features include weight loss, vomiting, diarrhoea, malaise, fever, vitiligo and muscle cramps. In females, loss of body hair occurs in both Addison's disease (due to loss of adrenal androgens) and secondary hypoadrenalism. In males, testicular androgens maintain body hair in Addison's disease.

Patients may also present with an Addisonian crisis. This is characterized by hypotension, hyponatraemia, hyperkalaemia, an elevated urea and a metabolic acidosis. Hypoglycaemia may also be present, though it is commoner with secondary hypoadrenalism caused by panhypopituitarism. Biochemistry may, however, be normal.

The causes of Addison's disease include:

1. Autoimmune destruction of the adrenal glands
2. Tuberculous destruction of the adrenal glands
3. Granulomatous infiltration
4. Metastatic carcinoma
5. Amyloidosis
6. Infarction of the adrenal cortex.

Adrenal insufficiency may be confirmed by:
- Measuring low plasma cortisol levels with no diurnal response and a raised plasma ACTH (raised in primary adrenal failure.)
- The short synacthen test: failure of plasma cortisol levels increase by at least 250 nmol/L to greater then 550 nmol/L.
- The long synacthen test can then be used to further confirm the diagnosis and distinguish between primary and secondary adrenal failure.

In a normal response	The plasma cortisol level would be expected to peak at 4 hours and not show a further response over 24 hours
In primary adrenal failure	The cortisol level will remain suppressed throughout the test
In secondary adrenal cortical failure	The plasma cortisol level increases throughout the test (because of residual function). The level at 24 hours is therefore greater then the 4-hour level

Other tests include:
- Measurement of adrenal antibodies
- Abdominal X-ray/CT imaging, which may show evidence of adrenal calcification with tuberculous adrenal destruction.

What is the diagnosis?

1. Cushing's syndrome
2. Addison's disease
3. Hypothyroidism
4. Graves' disease
5. Nephrotic syndrome

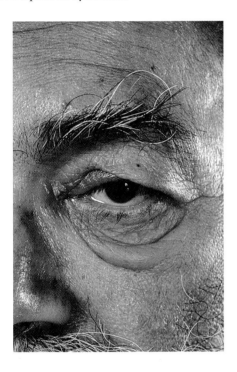

3. Hypothyroidism.

The slide shows thickened facial features associated with periorbital swelling. There is also loss of the outer third of the eyebrow. This is consistent with a diagnosis of hypothyroidism.

Common clinical features associated with **hypothyroidism** include:

General features:
Obesity
Goitre
Hyperlipidaemia
Myxoedematous facies: thickened and coarse facial features, periorbital puffiness and pallor
Skin is rough, dry, cold and inelastic with a yellow tinge (secondary to carotenaemia)
Generalized non-pitting swelling of the subcutaneous tissues
Thin, dry, brittle hair
Loss of outer third of eyebrows
Vitiligo
Alopecia
Menorrhagia and infertility
Anaemia
Gastrointestinal
Constipation
Ileus

Neuromuscular
Weakness: a painful proximal myopathy
Severe myalgia
Slow movements
Slow relaxing reflexes
Hoarse croaky voice
Carpal tunnel syndrome
Peripheral neuropathy
Deafness
Psychosis (myxoedema madness)
Depression
Hypersomnolence
Lethargy and mental slowing
Cerebellar signs

Cardiovascular
Angina
Bradycardia
Cardiac failure
Pleural/pericardial effusions

Other autoimmune diseases may also be present, these include:
Pernicious anaemia
Addison's disease
Vitiligo
Rheumatoid arthritis
Sjögren's syndrome
Ulcerative colitis
Chronic active hepatitis

SLE
Haemolytic anaemia
DM
Graves' disease
Hypoparathyroidism
Premature ovarian failure

The causes of hypothyroidism include:
- Primary:
  Iodine deficiency; Autoimmune diseases: Hashimoto's, primary myxoedema, atrophic thyroiditis; Iatrogenic: post-radiotherapy, post-surgery; Drugs: amiodarone, lithium, alpha-interferon, antithyroid drugs; Congenital: absent or ectopic gland/dyshormonogenesis; Destructive thyroiditis: post-partum, silent thyroiditis, de Quervain's thyroiditis; Infiltration: amyloid, sarcoid, Riedel's thyroiditis
- Secondary:
  Hypopituitarism, isolated TSH deficiency, hypothalamic disease.

This patient has been referred by the GP for further investigation of a possible cardiac murmur.

Which of the following is the most likely and significant cardiological abnormality in this patient?

1. Mitral valve disease
2. Hypertension
3. Tricuspid valve disease
4. Ventricular septal defect
5. Aortic valve disease

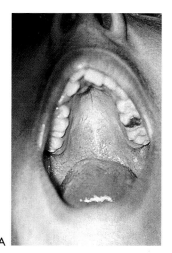
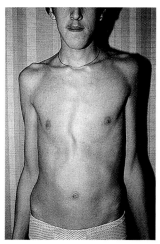

A   B

5. Aortic valve disease.

The slides show a high-arched palate and a depressed twisted sternum. The combination of these clinical features suggests a diagnosis of **Marfan's syndrome**. This is inherited as an autosomal dominant trait with variable penetrance. The defect is located in the fibrillin gene on chromosome 15. Fibrillin is particularly associated with elastin-containing tissues. This accounts for the commonest and most significant cardiological abnormality: dilation of the ascending aorta leading to aortic incompetence and dissection. Untreated these abnormalities are the leading cause of death.

Other clinical features include:
- Other cardiological complications: mitral valve prolapse, coarctation of the aorta, bacterial endocarditis
- Long, thin extremities with span greater than height
- Arachnodactyly
- Depressed, twisted sternum
- Spontaneous pneumothorax
- High-arched palate; scoliosis
- Upward dislocation of the lens*
- Joint and ligamentous laxity, osteoporosis
- Herniae.

*Note: Homocystinuria, an autosomal recessive inborn error of metabolism, is phenotypically similar to Marfan's syndrome. Clinical features of homocystinuria include: Marfanoid body habitus; downward dislocation of the lens; low IQ; osteoporosis; vascular thrombosis; and livedo reticularis. Cardiac complications do not occur in homocystinuria.

Which of the following is this patient most likely to develop?

1. Medullary cell carcinoma of the thyroid
2. Zollinger-Ellison Syndrome
3. Meningioma
4. Optic glioma
5. Pulmonary fibrosis

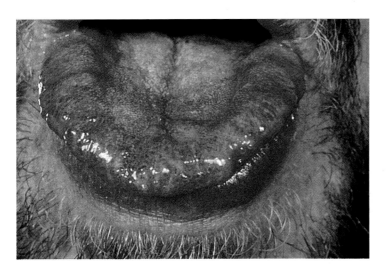

1. Medullary cell carcinoma of the thyroid.

The slide shows multiple mucosal neuromas of the tongue and lips. This patient has MEN IIB (multiple endocrine neoplasia) syndrome and medullary carcinoma of the thyroid invariably develops in such patients.

This syndrome is similar to MEN IIA (Sipple's syndrome: medullary cell carcinoma of the thyroid, phaeochromocytoma and parathyroid hyperplasia), but differs in that mucosal neuromas of the lips, cheeks and tongue are characteristic. Gastrointestinal ganglioneuromas, neuromas, neurofibromas, and café au lait spots may be also seen in MEN IIB and patients may also have a Marfanoid appearance. Inheritance is autosomal dominant, but is often sporadic. C-cell hyperplasia is found in 100% as in MEN IIA, and medullary thyroid cancer is seen in both. Parathyroid cell hyperplasia occurs in 80% of patients with MEN IIA, with symptomatic hypercalcaemia in 20%; hypercalcaemia is not a common feature of MEN IIB. The incidence of phaeochromocytoma is the same in MEN IIA and MEN IIB.

MEN I (Werner's syndrome) is characterized by parathyroid hyperplasia or adenomas (up to 95%), pancreatic adenoma in 70%, and pituitary adenoma in approximately 30%. Multiple lipomas are seen. Insulinomas are the most common pancreatic adenoma, but glucagonoma, gastrinoma (Zollinger–Ellison syndrome), somatostatinoma and serotoninoma have been described. Inheritance is autosomal dominant.

MEN I (AD)	Werner's syndrome	• Pituitary adenoma: detected in 30%, prolactinomas being the most common and acromegaly in a third • Parathyroid hyperplasia: hyperparathyroidism is the commonest presenting feature • Pancreatic endocrine tumours: pancreatic endocrine tumours occur in 70%; gastrinomas (Zollinger–Ellison) and insulinomas are the most common • Other features: multiple lipomas are also seen
MEN II (AD)	Sipple's	• Medullary cell carcinoma of the thyroid: tumour of thyroid C-cells; incidence 100%; total thyroidectomy is required • Phaeochromocytoma: occurs in 50% of cases • Other features: parathyroid hyperplasia in 80% but less then 20% have hypercalcaemia
MEN IIb (AD but 50% new mutations)	Sometimes referred to as MEN III	• Medullary cell carcinoma of the thyroid • Phaeochromocytoma • Marfanoid habitus and mucosal neuromata: neuromas are commonly ocular and oral

This 86-year-old female presented to casualty with a transient ischaemic attack and was found to be in atrial fibrillation. On routine clinical examination she was found to have a swollen right shoulder with marked restriction in the range of movement. Further questioning revealed she had fallen on to the right arm six months previously, since which she had lost mobility in the shoulder.

200 ml of blood-stained synovial fluid was aspirated and sent for analysis.

The likely diagnosis is:

1. Low-grade septic arthritis
2. Gout
3. Pseudogout
4. Hydroxyapatite arthritis
5. Cholesterol arthritis

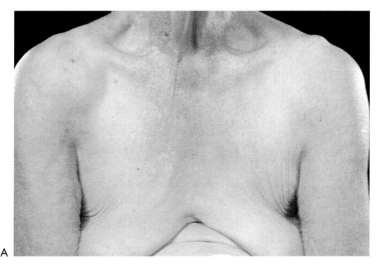

A

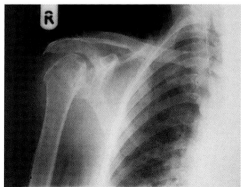

B

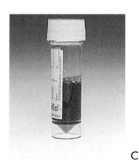

C

4. Hydroxyapatite arthritis.

A large right shoulder effusion is clearly visible. The plain X-ray shows severe destruction of the humeral head.

- The most likely diagnosis is Milwaukee shoulder. This often develops as a consequence of trauma, with degeneration of cartilage and shedding of hydroxyapatite crystals into the joint. Large shoulder effusions are typical and fluid aspirated is usually uniformly blood-stained. Alizarin red staining of the synovial fluid will demonstrate hydroxyapatite crystals and plain X-rays will show destruction of the humeral head.

The differential diagnosis includes sepsis and this always requires exclusion.

Appendix I Features of Systemic lupus erythematosus

Systemic lupus erythematosus is diagnosed if four or more of the following 11 features (*italics*) are present together or serially:

Malar rash	A fixed erythematous, flat or raised rash A classical butterfly rash found over the bridge of the nose and malar bones is present in two-thirds of patients
Discoid rash	Present in 15% of patients Erythematous raised patches with adherent keratotic scaling and follicular plugging; atrophic scarring may occur
Photosensitivity	Exposure to UV light causes the rash, accounting for its distribution over sun-exposed areas
Oral ulceration	Includes oral and nasopharyngeal ulceration Anorexia and abdominal pain can also occur Mucosal ulcers can become deep and infected with *Candida*
Arthritis	A non-erosive arthritis involving two or more peripheral joints, characterized by tenderness, swelling or effusion Musculoskeletal features affect more than 90% of patients
Serositis	Pleuritis or pericarditis documented by ECG or rub or evidence of a pericardial effusion Pulmonary disease occurs in 40%; common manifestations are pleurisy or small pleural effusions Parenchymal involvement is rare Pericarditis is more common then myocarditis and patients can also develop an endocarditis (Libman–Sacks endocarditis)
Renal	• Proteinuria >0.5 g/24 hours or 3+ persistently or • Cellular casts
Neurological	Seizures or psychosis without evidence of another cause Almost any neurological abnormality can be present
Haematological	• Haemolytic anaemia or • Leukopenia < 4.0×10^9 on two or more separate occasions or • Lymphopenia < 1.5×10^9 on two or more occasions • Thrombocytopenia < 100×10^9 A normochromic haemolytic anaemia is present in 70% and there is also commonly a Coombs-positive haemolytic anaemia

Immunological	• Raised anti-ds DNA antibody binding or
	• Anti-Sm antibody or
	• Positive finding of antiphospholipid antibodies based on:
	  – An abnormal level of serum IgG or IgM anticardiolipin antibodies
	  – A positive test for the lupus anticoagulant
	A false positive serological test for syphilis, present for a least six months

Anti-nuclear antibody in raised titre	An abnormal titre of ANA, in the absence of drugs known to induce ANAs

INDEX

NB: *Numbers in the index refer to questions not pages.*

INDEX